Clinical Oral Pathology

Nabil Kochaji

Clinical Oral Pathology

Kochaji's Guide to Oral Lesions and Biopsies

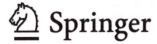

Nabil Kochaji
Oral Histology and Pathology
Damascus University-Faculty of Dentistry
Damascus, Syrian Arab Republic

ISBN 978-3-031-53754-7   ISBN 978-3-031-53755-4   (eBook)
https://doi.org/10.1007/978-3-031-53755-4

© The Editor(s) (if applicable) and The Author(s), under exclusive license to Springer Nature Switzerland AG 2024

This work is subject to copyright. All rights are solely and exclusively licensed by the Publisher, whether the whole or part of the material is concerned, specifically the rights of translation, reprinting, reuse of illustrations, recitation, broadcasting, reproduction on microfilms or in any other physical way, and transmission or information storage and retrieval, electronic adaptation, computer software, or by similar or dissimilar methodology now known or hereafter developed.

The use of general descriptive names, registered names, trademarks, service marks, etc. in this publication does not imply, even in the absence of a specific statement, that such names are exempt from the relevant protective laws and regulations and therefore free for general use.

The publisher, the authors, and the editors are safe to assume that the advice and information in this book are believed to be true and accurate at the date of publication. Neither the publisher nor the authors or the editors give a warranty, expressed or implied, with respect to the material contained herein or for any errors or omissions that may have been made. The publisher remains neutral with regard to jurisdictional claims in published maps and institutional affiliations.

This Springer imprint is published by the registered company Springer Nature Switzerland AG
The registered company address is: Gewerbestrasse 11, 6330 Cham, Switzerland

Paper in this product is recyclable.

Preface

The health and aesthetics of the dental arch are of paramount importance to both the dentist and the patient in daily dental care. Regrettably, oral lesions often take a backseat, being addressed as secondary concerns or sometimes even later.

Sentences like:

– "A radiolucent lesion attached to the apex of a non-vital tooth is either a Periapical Granuloma or a Radicular Cyst, and nothing more."
– "A radiolucent lesion surrounding an impacted tooth is always an innocent Dentigerous Cyst."

often linger in the minds of the majority of dentists, especially general practitioners, who unfortunately may be assigning these incorrect roles when dealing with patients.

This issue diminishes the patient's likelihood of early lesion diagnosis and could potentially squander crucial time. Furthermore, it carries the risk of a significant catastrophe, such as substantial loss of oral tissues.

The forthcoming guidelines encapsulate the distilled wisdom garnered from 17 years of professional oral maxillofacial pathology practice, as well as the ongoing management of thousands of cases attended to in the clinics of numerous dentists. My aspiration is that these insights prove valuable in enhancing comprehension of Clinical Oral Pathology, ultimately translating into more effective treatment for all our patients.

The first volume will focus on intraosseous lesions, while the second volume will delve into oral mucosal lesions. Throughout both volumes, emphasis will be placed on clinical and radiographic features. While histological characteristics undeniably play a pivotal role in establishing the ultimate diagnosis, their discussion will be limited to the essential, as they stand further removed from a doctor's day-to-day practice within their clinic.

The majority of the book will adopt either a question-and-answer format or a bullet-point structure. My intention is to steer clear of using purely pathological terminology and instead prioritize the language commonly used in everyday clinical practice.

While certain guides and advantages may appear highly simplified, this approach is intentional, driven by the ultimate goal of making the text accessible and beneficial to a wide audience.

You might see from a quick reading a lot of repeated ideas; in fact each time a lesion was repeated it was for a new purpose, it's just a story book, story that every dental practitioner can and should read far away from books addressed to scholars and academics!

With 93 tips, more than 70 cases which I followed, sectioned and through my microscope lens analyzed.

I wish that this book would be a cross-road and that your dental practice to Clinical Oral Pathology would never be the same after reading it!

Damascus, Syrian Arab Republic   Nabil Kochaji
18/12/2022

Contents

1 Oral Maxillofacial Biopsies 1
  1.1 Preface 1
      1.1.1 What Is Pathology? 1
      1.1.2 Is Pathology One Specialty? 1
      1.1.3 Do we Always Need a Pathological Study? 2
      1.1.4 When Does Oral Pathology Start to Be a
           Distinguished Dental Specialty? 3
      1.1.5 Should We Take the Consultation of the Oral and
           Maxillofacial Pathologist in Particular? 4
  1.2 Introductory Guides in Oral Biopsies 5
      1.2.1 Why Do We Need (Oral) Pathology in Everyday
           Practice? 5
      1.2.2 When to Decide to Perform Biopsy? 8
      1.2.3 What Types of Biopsies a Dentist Can Perform? 11
      1.2.4 Factors Influencing the Type of Biopsy Selection 12
      1.2.5 How to Handle and Transport Biopsy? 13
      1.2.6 What Is the Fluid with which to Transport the Biopsy
           to the Pathology Lab? 15
      1.2.7 How to Deal with the Oral Pathologist 20
      1.2.8 Gross Pathology (Specimen Macropathology
           Examination) 25
      1.2.9 Histological Preparation of a Specimen 29
      1.2.10 Histological Findings 30
      1.2.11 How Do We Read the Histopathology Report? 35
      1.2.12 How to Read the Final Result from Pathological Report? ... 39
      1.2.13 How to Benefit from Recommendations Section 46
  References 47

2 Intraosseous Lesions 49
  2.1 General Algorism 49
  2.2 Differential Diagnosis of a Unilocular Radiolucent Lesion
    in the Jaws (Algorithm of Logic Thinking) 52
      2.2.1 Introduction 52

vii

	2.2.2	Top Differential Diagnosis for Unilocular Radiolucent Lesion	52
	2.2.3	Algorithm for Differential Diagnosis.	55
	2.2.4	Vital Teeth	56
	2.2.5	Nonvital Teeth	61
	2.2.6	Edentulous Area.	65
	2.2.7	Impacted Tooth	67
2.3		Differential Diagnosis of a Multilocular Radiolucent Lesion in the Jaws (Algorithm of Logic Thinking).	68
	2.3.1	Introduction	68
	2.3.2	Top Differential Diagnosis for Multilocular Radiolucent Lesion	69
	2.3.3	Algorithm for Differential Diagnosis.	71
	2.3.4	Vital Teeth	72
	2.3.5	Nonvital Teeth	73
	2.3.6	Edentulous Area.	75
	2.3.7	Located Near an Impacted Tooth.	78
2.4		Differential Diagnosis of a Radiopaque Lesion in the Jaws (Algorithm of Logic Thinking)	78
	2.4.1	Introduction	78
	2.4.2	Top Common Radiopaque Lesions	78
	2.4.3	Algorithm for Differential Diagnosis.	81
2.5		Categorization and Comprehensive Classification of Intraosseous Radiopaque Lesions in the Jaws	83
	2.5.1	Benign Neoplastic Lesions	83
	2.5.2	Fibro-Osseous Lesions.	84
	2.5.3	Metabolic and Systemic Conditions	84
	2.5.4	Malignant Lesions	85
	2.5.5	Developmental and Anatomical Variants.	85
	2.5.6	Vital Teeth	86
	2.5.7	Nonvital Teeth	87
	2.5.8	Edentulous Area.	88
2.6		Differential Diagnosis of a Mixed Radiolucent/Radiopaque Lesion in the Jaws (Algorithm of Logic Thinking)	89
	2.6.1	Introduction	89
	2.6.2	Top Frequent Mixed Lesions	89
	2.6.3	Algorithm for Differential Diagnosis.	90
	2.6.4	Vital Teeth	91
	2.6.5	Nonvital Teeth	92
	2.6.6	Edentulous Area.	92
2.7		Summary of Part Two	92
	2.7.1	Lesion Seen on Radiographs as a Unilocular Radiolucent Lesion on an Erupted and Vital Tooth	93
	2.7.2	Lesion Seen on Radiographs as a Unilocular Radiolucent Lesion on a Nonerupted Tooth	94
References.			95

Contents

3 All Intraosseous Lesion of the Jaws 97
  3.1 Odontogenic Cysts............................. 97
    3.1.1 Introduction 97
    3.1.2 Definition of Odontogenic Cysts 98
    3.1.3 Importance in Dentistry and Oral Medicine 98
    3.1.4 Classification of Odontogenic Cysts 99
    3.1.5 Etiology and Pathogenesis........................ 100
    3.1.6 Cyst Formation and Growing....................... 101
    3.1.7 Radiographic and Histological Features 101
    3.1.8 Clinical Presentation 102
    3.1.9 Radiographic Findings......................... 103
    3.1.10 Differential Diagnosis 104
    3.1.11 Final Diagnosis 104
    3.1.12 Management and Treatment....................... 104
    3.1.13 Management of Recurrent Cysts 105
    3.1.14 Adjunctive Therapies (e.g., Carnoy's Solution)........... 105
    3.1.15 Follow-Up and Monitoring 106
    3.1.16 Complications and Their Management 106
    3.1.17 Prognosis and Long-Term Outcomes................... 107
    3.1.18 Odontogenic Cysts in Pediatric Dentistry 107
    3.1.19 Prevention and Future Directions 108
    3.1.20 Conclusion........................... 108
  3.2 Non-odontogenic Cysts 109
    3.2.1 Introduction 109
    3.2.2 Definition of Non-odontogenic Cysts 109
    3.2.3 Importance in Dentistry and Oral Medicine 110
    3.2.4 Classification of Odontogenic Cysts 110
    3.2.5 Etiology and Pathogenesis........................ 110
    3.2.6 Clinical Presentation 110
    3.2.7 Diagnosis 110
    3.2.8 Management and Treatment....................... 111
    3.2.9 Complications and Their Management 111
    3.2.10 Conclusion........................... 111
  3.3 Odontogenic Tumors 111
    3.3.1 Introduction 111
    3.3.2 Definition of Odontogenic Tumors 111
    3.3.3 Importance in Dentistry and Oral Medicine 112
    3.3.4 Classification of Odontogenic Tumors.................. 112
    3.3.5 Etiology and Pathogenesis........................ 113
    3.3.6 Clinical Presentation 113
    3.3.7 Diagnosis 113
    3.3.8 Management and Treatment....................... 114
    3.3.9 Complications and Their Management 114
    3.3.10 Prognosis and Long-Term Outcomes................... 114
    3.3.11 Conclusion........................... 115

3.4 Non-odontogenic Tumors 115
    3.4.1 Introduction 115
    3.4.2 Definition of Non-odontogenic Tumors. 115
    3.4.3 Importance in Dentistry and Oral Medicine 115
    3.4.4 Classification of Non-odontogenic Tumors 116
    3.4.5 Etiology and Pathogenesis. 117
    3.4.6 Clinical Presentation 117
    3.4.7 Diagnosis 118
    3.4.8 Management and Treatment. 118
    3.4.9 Management of Recurrent Tumors 119
    3.4.10 Follow-Up and Monitoring 119
    3.4.11 Complications and Their Management 120
    3.4.12 Prognosis and Long-Term Outcomes. 121
    3.4.13 Conclusion 121
3.5 Intraosseous Primary Malignancies. 121
    3.5.1 Introduction 121
    3.5.2 Importance in Dentistry and Oral Medicine 121
    3.5.3 Classification of Primary Intraosseous Malignancies 123
    3.5.4 Etiology and Pathogenesis. 123
    3.5.5 Clinical Presentation 124
    3.5.6 Differential Diagnosis 125
    3.5.7 Diagnosis 126
    3.5.8 Management and Treatment. 127
    3.5.9 Management of Recurrent Malignancies. 127
    3.5.10 Complications and Their Management 127
    3.5.11 Prognosis and Long-Term Outcomes. 130
    3.5.12 Conclusion 131
3.6 Intraosseous Secondary (Metastatic) Malignancies. 132
    3.6.1 Introduction 132
    3.6.2 Importance in Dentistry and Oral Medicine 132
    3.6.3 Classification of Primary Malignancies. 133
    3.6.4 Etiology and Pathogenesis. 134
    3.6.5 Clinical Presentation 135
    3.6.6 Diagnosis 136
    3.6.7 Management and Treatment. 138
    3.6.8 Management of Recurrent Malignancies. 138
    3.6.9 Follow-Up and Monitoring 140
    3.6.10 Complications and Their Management 142
    3.6.11 Prognosis and Long-Term Outcomes. 142
    3.6.12 Conclusion 142
References. 142

4 General Benefits 145
4.1 Can Radicular Cysts Be Healed by Endodontic Treatment? 145
4.2 Algorithms for Dealing with Unilocular Radiolucent Lesion 147
    4.2.1 Algorithm for Managing Unilocular Radiolucent Lesions .. 147

	4.3	Four Main Lesions That a Dentist May Encounter Frequently in Daily Dental Practice	148
		4.3.1 Radicular Cyst	148
		4.3.2 Dentigerous Cyst	151
		4.3.3 Odontogenic Keratocyst	154
		4.3.4 Ameloblastoma	157
	4.4	Are Rare Lesions Really Rare?	160
	4.5	Short Stories	163
		4.5.1 The Painful Sorrow	163
		4.5.2 The Mysterious Lesion	164
		4.5.3 The Hidden Threat	165
	4.6	Catastrophic True Case	166
	References		167

Index 169

List of Figures

Fig. 1.1 (Benefit of biopsy) Each sample excised from the human body must undergo histological examination to determine: the type of disease and its pathogenesis → accurate diagnosis → optimal treatment → knowing the duration of follow-up (if necessary) → cure.................................... 9

Fig. 1.2 (Excisonal biopsy) Small soft tissue lesion in the palate; the decision should be excisional biopsy..................... 13

Fig. 1.3 (Incisional biopsy) Large soft tissue lesion in the palate; the decision should be incisional biopsy..................... 13

Fig. 1.4 Amount of fixative liquid. (**a**) The specimen. (**b**) Less than adequate immersing in fixative solution. (**c**) Best amount. (**d**) More than enough 15

Fig. 1.5 Making incisions in the sample mass using a surgical scalpel 18

Fig. 1.6 Rinsing the fresh sample in saline.......................... 20

Fig. 1.7 The surgical report template. Frontal page: (documentation)..... 21

Fig. 1.8 The surgical report template. Back page: (orientation).......... 22

Fig. 1.9 Orienting the biopsy using surgical sutures................... 25

Fig. 1.10 Specimen measurement.................................. 26

Fig. 1.11 Specimen weight....................................... 26

Fig. 1.12 Gross pathology and sample sectioning. When dissecting the lesion attached to the impacted third molar, it was found to be a cystic lesion. Subsequently, histological examination confirmed it to be a unicystic ameloblastoma 27

Fig. 1.13 Gross pathology and sample sectioning. In another lesion with a similar clinical impression and radiographic features, the macroscopic examination revealed a solid mass rather than a cystic appearance, the final diagnosis was odontogenic myxoma... 28

Fig. 1.14 Gross pathology and sample sectioning. Revealing the cystic structure of the lesion 28

Fig. 1.15 Gross pathology and sample sectioning. Exploring the complete loss of normal maxillary osseous structure and the different coloration of the sectioned area........................... 29

Fig. 1.16	Histological view of radicular cyst. Same case as shown in Fig. 1.14.	31
Fig. 1.17	Routine H&E staining, IHC staining. (**a**) Routine H&E staining (left). (**b**) Same histological section with CD20 IHC staining to show B-lymphocytes (right)	32
Fig. 1.18	SCC histological grading. Three cases of squamous cell carcinoma, from left to right: well, moderate, and poorly differentiated	32
Fig. 1.19	Odontogenic keratocyst histological features. Both cases are OKC. (**a**) (case 1): Without epithelial separation. (**b**) (case 2): With epithelial separation, which increases the probability of recurrence. (**c**) (case 2): Daughter cyst also increases the probability of recurrence	35
Fig. 1.20	Histological patterns of SCC invasion. Both cases are SCC. (**a**) Invasion pattern is bushing. (**b**): Invasion pattern is penetrating, which increases the probability of recurrence	35
Fig. 1.21	Periapical granuloma cases. To the left presence of rests of Malassez, to the right: absence of rests of Malassez.	36
Fig. 1.22	Dentigerous cyst cases. To the left: presence of rests of mucus cells; to the right: absence of mucus cells	36
Fig. 1.23	Ameloblastoma cases	37
Fig. 1.24	First page of the pathological report of a case of ameloblastoma. Unfortunately, the patient himself is a 23-year-old dentist!	42
Fig. 1.25	Second page of the same pathological report of Fig. 1.24. It shows the exact subtype of ameloblastoma	43
Fig. 1.26	Two cases of odontogenic keratocyst. The first (upper) was treated in a manner time; the second (down) suffered from four recurrences and ended in semi-mandibular ectomy!.	47
Fig. 2.1	Radiolucent lesion in the left mandibular body causing clinical swelling, attached to nonvital primary molars, and containing impacted premolars	51
Fig. 2.2	Macro and micro view for the case shown in Fig. 2.1. It turned out to be a radicular cyst	52
Fig. 2.3	Two symmetric impacted third molars, associated with unilocular radiolucent lesions	54
Fig. 2.4	Lesions shown in Fig. 2.3. Both lesions were cystic; still, the right one was dentigerous and the left was odontogenic keratocyst!	54
Fig. 2.5	Radiolucent lesion on an impacted third molar. This unilocular radiolucent lesion surrounding the impacted third molar looks like an innocent dentigerous cyst only!.	56
Fig. 2.6	Macroscopic study for the lesion in Fig. 2.5. Macroscopically, it is attached to the neck of the impacted teeth; still, when sectioning, it was solid rather than cystic	57

Fig. 2.7	The histopathological view of the lesion in Figs. 2.5 and 2.6. Finally, it turned out to be odontogenic myxoma!.	57
Fig. 2.8	Radiolucent lesion on vital molar. This molar with acute pulpitis symptoms cannot make a radicular cyst; still, the radiolucency exists!	58
Fig. 2.9	Macroscopic analysis of the lesion in Fig. 2.8. Macroscopic examination showed tiny fragments without specific notable observation.	58
Fig. 2.10	The histopathological view of lesions appeared in Figs. 2.8 and 2.9. Finally, it was proven histologically to be an aneurysmal bone cyst. The case should be before pulp symptoms appear, but there was no radiographic history available with the patient	59
Fig. 2.11	Radiolucency appeared at the apex of the first mandibular molar. The only question mark was that teeth is vital; otherwise, the dentist would call it a radicular cyst only!	59
Fig. 2.12	Macroscopic analysis of the lesion in Fig. 2.11. Macroscopically, it was fragmented and could never be enucleated as a one-piece specimen; that was another sign. The third was clear upon sectioning: the metallic feeling!	60
Fig. 2.13	The histopathological view of the lesion in Figs. 2.11 and 2.12. On histopathological study, the case was diagnosed as ossifying fibroma.	60
Fig. 2.14	Well-defined unilocular radiolucency at the apex of nonvital canine and poorly treated premolar	61
Fig. 2.15	Macroscopic and microscopic analyses of the lesion in Fig. 2.14. Macroscopically, it was proven to be a cystic lesion; microscopically, it was a radicular cyst	62
Fig. 2.16	Typical radiographic appearance of a radicular cyst	62
Fig. 2.17	Macroscopic and microscopic analyses of the lesion in Fig. 2.16. Macroscopically, it was proven to be a cystic lesion; microscopically, it was a radicular cyst	63
Fig. 2.18	Clinical and radiographic appearance of a case of CGCG. Although peripheral giant cell granuloma is a gingival rather than intraosseous disease, it can make a fingerprint on the underlined jaws.	64
Fig. 2.19	Post-operation specimen. Wide excision to reach the osseous part is essential to minimize recurrence	64
Fig. 2.20	Histopathological view of a case in Figs. 2.18 and 2.19. Just beneath the epithelium, we can see hemosiderin spots due to masticatory forces against the gingiva, and far away the multinucleated giant cells are easily seen	65
Fig. 2.21	Impacted canine surrounded by a radiolucent unilocular lesion	67

Fig. 2.22	Macroscopic and microscopic analysis of the lesion in Fig. 2.21. Nothing important was visible on macroscopic study, no sectioning clear cystic structure was detected, and histological examination proved OKC case	67
Fig. 2.23	Radiolucent lesion distal of the third mandibular molar. Occasionally in the retromolar area some ectopic minor salivary glands might be detected	68
Fig. 2.24	Multilocular radiolucent lesion	69
Fig. 2.25	Histological view of the lesion in Fig. 2.24. Histologically, it was proven to be OKC, having all alarms of high recurrence rates, epithelial separation, and daughter cysts	70
Fig. 2.26	Multilocular radiolucent lesion in the anterior mandible. This huge radiolucent multilocular lesion was thought as a dentigerous cyst, and a marsupialization was scheduled. The incisional biopsy proved it was a cystic lesion.	71
Fig. 2.27	Glandular odontogenic cyst.	73
Fig. 2.28	Soup bubble multilocular radiolucent lesion.	74
Fig. 2.29	Same case as of Fig. 2.27. The diagnosis is conventional ameloblastoma.	74
Fig. 2.30	Multilocular radiolucent/mixed lesion in the maxilla. A 2-year delay in diagnosing the case cost this 45-year-old lady the loss of her jaw	75
Fig. 2.31	The case of Fig. 2.30. It was finally diagnosed as a Pindborg tumor	76
Fig. 2.32	3D and histological view of a sad case. This central giant cell tumor was treated as an abscess for several months!	76
Fig. 2.33	Odontoma development through a 3-year period	77
Fig. 2.34	Macroscopic examination of the case of odontoma. Macroscopically, the specimen was very hard; using nitric acid gave the specimen this yellow color	79
Fig. 2.35	Histopathological features of odontoma. Irregular dentin tubules of complex odontoma	79
Fig. 2.36	Case of recurrent osteoma	80
Fig. 2.37	Osteomyelitis on a patient under bisphosphonate treatment	81
Fig. 2.38	Osteoma case	82
Fig. 2.39	Case of fibrous dysplasia, discovered accidentally on a radiograph	84
Fig. 2.40	Bilateral ossifying fibroma	85
Fig. 2.41	Delay of diagnosis of Pindborg tumor.	91
Fig. 2.42	A lesion that was frequently described as a residual cyst turned out to be a plasmacytoma!	93
Fig. 3.1	Radiolucent lesion attached to impacted teeth. It looks like an innocent dentigerous cyst, on radiographs and even on macroscopic sectioning, but it is in fact glandular odontogenic cyst	100

Fig. 3.2	A radiolucent lesion associated with impacted third molar. It could be any developmental odontogenic cyst or tumor. In this case final diagnosis was odontogenic keratocyst	102
Fig. 3.3	Patient suffered from pathological fracture due to non-treated residual cyst	106
Fig. 3.4	Radiolucent lesion in the mandibular angle. Although it looks on radiographs and by macroscopic sectioning as a primordial cyst	107
Fig. 3.5	Histopathological view of lesion in Fig. 3.4. The serial sectioning showed a benign neoplastic transformation in the epithelial cystic lining	107
Fig. 3.6	Two images for the same odontogenic cyst. Note that in CT scan image the cortical bone was expanded and preserved, and not penetrated, while 3D CBCT showed an illusion of cortical bone penetration	108
Fig. 3.7	Case of ossifying fibroma	120
Fig. 3.8	Fibrosarcoma detailed case. This poor lady, 52 years old, suffered from fibrosarcoma, the late diagnosis was mainly due to thoughts that it can be an odontogenic tumor, and there is no need to further evaluation; after final diagnosis was established, cervical nodule involvement was discovered, and neck dissection operation was performed	128
Fig. 4.1	Radicular cyst case. On radiograph, look how it preserved cortical bone, and the mandibular alveolar nerve	149
Fig. 4.2	Dentigerous cyst case. Old theory that distinguishes between dentigerous cyst and dilated dental follicle depending on radiographs can be proven wrong with this case of dentigerous cyst	152
Fig. 4.3	Dentigerous cyst case. The patient came with the chief complaint of acute pulpal pain from the second molar; it's obvious that the impacted third molar and its dentigerous cyst are the cause	152
Fig. 4.4	Odontogenic keratocyst case. On radiograph, macroscopically and upon sectioning it looks like dentigerous cyst, still the microscope lens has another point of view with this odontogenic keratocyst	155
Fig. 4.5	Ameloblastoma case. The red lines were drawn by the oral maxillofacial surgeon who performed the resection of this case of recurrent ameloblastoma	157
Fig. 4.6	Case of ossifying fibroma on an implant	161
Fig. 4.7	Case of squamous cell carcinoma	166

About the Author

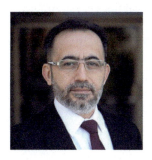

Nabil Kochaji
Work Experience
Member of WHO-AI group of Oral Maxillofacial Cancers (2022)
Founding Dean, faculty of dentistry, Al-Sham Private University (2016–2019)
Head of Oral Pathology and Histology Department, Damascus University (2010–2014)
Founding and running first and only oral maxillofacial pathology service in the Middle East (since 2005)
Prof. of Oral Histology, Oral Pathology in Damascus University (since 2005)

Awards
Senior Robert Frank Award Holder, International Association of Dental Research (IADR), the Netherlands (2005)

Degrees
Doctor in Dentistry from Damascus University (Syria) (1997)
Master's in Medical and Pharmaceutical Research from Brussels University, Belgium (2002)
PhD in Dentistry from Brussels University, Belgium (2005)

Membership
President: Syrian National Board of Oral Maxillofacial Pathology (2021)
President: Syrian National Society of Oral Pathology (2019)
Secretary General: Syrian National Board of Forensic Medicine (2014)
Member of the Syrian Society of Oncology (2007)
Member of the Belgian Royal Society of Pathologists (2002)
Member of the International Academy of Pathology, western Europe Division (2002)

Publishing Experience
Co-publisher and translator for Medical titles with Elsevier (since 2010)
Book Authorship
Author of 17 published medical titles (14 in Arabic, 3 translated) (since 2007)
Co-author of *Contemporary Oral Medicine* (Springer) (2017)
Author of three novels published in two languages (science fiction and thriller) (2014–2016–2019)

Oral Maxillofacial Biopsies

1

1.1 Preface

These guides will commence with an intellectual and philosophical introduction, aimed at extracting the utmost benefit from this specialization within the dentist's practice. These introductory concepts will be presented in a question-and-answer format:

1.1.1 What Is Pathology?

The Greek word "pathology" comprises two syllables: "Patho," signifying "Pain," which subsequently evolved to represent "Disease." This term extended into Latin as "pathologia" and then made its way into English, French, and German as "pathology," "pathologie," and "Pathologie," respectively. From this root, the word "patient," meaning the same in most languages of Latin origin, also emerged [1].

The term then transitioned to its new meaning, representing the "*Study of Diseases*" [2].

1.1.2 Is Pathology One Specialty?

Pathology is a diverse and indispensable field of medical science that focuses on the study of disease processes [1]. It holds a pivotal role in comprehending the fundamental mechanisms of illnesses, facilitating precise diagnoses, and shaping successful treatment approaches. While often thought of as a singular specialty, pathology actually encompasses various subdisciplines, each delving into unique facets of disease assessment [2].

© The Author(s), under exclusive license to Springer Nature Switzerland AG 2024
N. Kochaji, *Clinical Oral Pathology*,
https://doi.org/10.1007/978-3-031-53755-4_1

Pathology Subspecialties:

1. **Anatomical Pathology:** Often referred to as *surgical pathology*, anatomical pathology entails the microscopic evaluation of tissues and cells to diagnose diseases. Pathologists within this domain analyze biopsies and surgical samples, pinpointing irregularities that could suggest cancer, inflammation, infections, or other pathologic states. Anatomical pathology offers invaluable perspectives on disease classification, prognosis, and treatment choices.
2. **Clinical Pathology:** Referred to as *laboratory medicine* or *clinical laboratory science*, clinical pathology centers on scrutinizing bodily fluids and other samples to offer diagnostic insights. This subfield encompasses hematology, clinical chemistry, microbiology, immunology, and molecular diagnostics. Clinical pathologists hold a significant role in interpreting laboratory findings, contributing to the identification, tracking, and treatment of diverse medical conditions.
3. **Cytopathology:** Cytopathology involves the examination of cells shed or aspirated from body surfaces or fluids. Pathologists in this field assess cells for signs of malignancy or other pathological changes. Cytopathology is commonly used for cancer screening (e.g., Pap smears for cervical cancer) and the diagnosis of conditions affecting organs such as the thyroid, breast, and pancreas.
4. **Hematopathology:** Hematopathology deals with the study of blood disorders, including various types of leukemia, lymphomas, and other hematological malignancies. Hematopathologists analyze blood smears, bone marrow aspirates, and lymph node biopsies to diagnose and classify blood-related diseases accurately.
5. **Dermatopathology:** Dermatopathology focuses on the examination of skin biopsies to diagnose skin diseases and disorders. Dermatopathologists combine expertise in dermatology and pathology to accurately identify skin conditions, including inflammatory dermatoses, skin cancers, and autoimmune disorders.
6. **Neuropathology:** Neuropathology is concerned with the diagnosis of diseases affecting the nervous system, including the brain and spinal cord. Neuropathologists study brain biopsies, autopsies, and neurosurgical specimens to diagnose conditions such as brain tumors, neurodegenerative diseases, and infections [3].

1.1.3 Do we Always Need a Pathological Study?

The general rule says:

> (Tip 1): Every surgically removed portion of the human body necessitates a histopathological evaluation. The oral cavity stands as no exception to this imperative.

Nonetheless, this rule warrants comprehensive clarification. While pathological examinations hold a pivotal role in diagnosing and comprehending diverse diseases and conditions, their indispensability might not extend to every clinical circumstance. The necessity for a pathological analysis hinges on multiple aspects, encompassing the character of the patient's symptoms, their medical background, and the discretion of the healthcare practitioner.

In numerous instances, a clinical assessment harmonized with *noninvasive diagnostic methods*, like imaging investigations or laboratory assessments, might yield ample data to formulate a diagnosis and steer treatment determinations. For prevalent conditions characterized by clearly defined diagnostic criteria and foreseeable clinical manifestations, the routine necessity of a pathological analysis might be obviated.

Nevertheless, there exist scenarios where a pathological examination becomes imperative. Some instances in which a pathological study is often essential include:

1. **Uncertain or Complex Diagnoses:** When the clinical display is unusual or the diagnosis remains ambiguous, a pathological analysis can supply supplementary insights to validate or refine the diagnosis. This is particularly pertinent for infrequent or exceptional conditions.
2. **Suspected Malignancies:** Pathological scrutiny of tissue specimens is indispensable for diagnosing and gauging the extent of cancers. It facilitates the determination of tumor type, grade, and magnitude, pivotal factors in devising treatment strategies and forecasting outcomes.
3. **Monitoring Disease Evolution and Treatment Response:** Pathological analyses may prove indispensable in gauging treatment effectiveness, tracking disease advancement, or evaluating the reaction to therapy over time. This holds notable significance for persistent or progressive diseases.
4. **Research Aims:** Pathological inquiries contribute to medical research by furnishing insights into disease mechanisms, probing novel treatments, and devising predictive markers. They wield a pivotal role in advancing medical knowledge and enhancing patient care.

1.1.4 When Does Oral Pathology Start to Be a Distinguished Dental Specialty?

With the advancement of medical sciences and the expansion of their specializations, dentistry became an independent branch from the study of human medicine, although they still share a medical stem of basic sciences.

Then, specialization became a distinguished feature of the era and civilizational development, so the doctor studied surgery and the dentist studied the same surgical principles and then applied them in one of the most complex anatomical places and innovates! A doctor specializes in pediatrics, while a pediatric dentist focuses on treating children's dental health after studying the same fundamental aspects of psychology, child development, growth, and pediatric diseases.

Oral and maxillofacial pathology has naturally evolved into a distinct and dedicated specialization, requiring individuals holding dentistry degrees to undertake its study. This positioning renders oral pathologists exceptionally adept at interacting with dentists of various specializations and equips them to provide precise diagnoses while navigating the intricate landscape of the oral cavity and its adjacent regions [4].

It is important to acknowledge that their education entails mastering both histological and anatomical principles, alongside retaining a firm grasp of the fundamental tenets of pathology.

1.1.5   Should We Take the Consultation of the Oral and Maxillofacial Pathologist in Particular?

The answer is in one word, yes and certainly as far as we can reach one!

The examples of this are countless, they are benefits, tips, and guidelines in themselves, and I will list some of them in successive paragraphs.

When it comes to diagnosing and managing oral and maxillofacial diseases, including oral pathology, consulting with an oral and maxillofacial pathologist is highly beneficial and often recommended. Oral and maxillofacial pathologists specialize in the diagnosis of diseases specifically affecting the oral and maxillofacial region, including the oral cavity, jaws, salivary glands, and adjacent structures.

Here are some reasons why consulting an oral and maxillofacial pathologist can be advantageous:

1. **Expertise in oral and maxillofacial pathology:**
   Oral and maxillofacial pathologists undergo specialized training and education focused on the study of diseases and conditions specific to the oral and maxillofacial region. They possess in-depth knowledge of oral diseases, including their histopathological characteristics, clinical correlations, and treatment implications.
2. **Familiarity with oral disease spectrum:**
   Oral and maxillofacial pathologists have extensive experience in evaluating a wide range of oral conditions, including oral cancers, precancerous lesions, oral manifestations of systemic diseases, and odontogenic and nonodontogenic cysts and tumors. They are well-versed in recognizing and interpreting the microscopic features of these conditions, which aids in accurate diagnosis and appropriate treatment planning.
3. **Specialized diagnostic techniques:**
   Oral and maxillofacial pathologists are skilled in employing specific diagnostic techniques relevant to oral pathology, such as immunohistochemistry, special stains, and molecular diagnostics. These techniques can provide additional information about the nature, behavior, and prognosis of certain oral diseases, enhancing the precision of diagnosis and aiding in personalized treatment decisions.

4. **Collaboration with other specialists:**

Oral and maxillofacial pathologists often work closely with other dental and medical specialists, including oral and maxillofacial surgeons, dentists, oncologists, and radiologists, as part of a multidisciplinary team. Their expertise and input contribute to comprehensive patient care, treatment planning, and follow-up.

> (Tip 2): While general pathologists are trained in various aspects of pathology, including oral pathology, their scope of practice typically extends beyond the oral and maxillofacial region. In complex or challenging cases specific to the oral cavity or maxillofacial area, consulting an oral and maxillofacial pathologist can provide a more specialized and focused evaluation.

It is worth noting that the involvement of both general pathologists and oral and maxillofacial pathologists can be valuable in certain scenarios, promoting collaboration and knowledge exchange between the two distinct specialties. The specific circumstances and complexity of the case, as well as the availability of specialists, may influence the decision to involve an oral and maxillofacial pathologist.

Ultimately, consulting with an oral and maxillofacial pathologist can provide specialized expertise and enhance the accuracy of diagnosis and treatment planning for oral and maxillofacial diseases.

1.2 Introductory Guides in Oral Biopsies

1.2.1 Why Do We Need (Oral) Pathology in Everyday Practice?

It is important to note that the decision to pursue a pathological study is made by healthcare professionals (in the case of everyday dental practice, it is the dentists) based on the individual patient's circumstances. They consider various factors, including clinical findings, diagnostic uncertainty, potential benefits, and risks associated with the procedure. The ultimate goal is to provide the most accurate diagnosis and appropriate management for the patient's specific condition.

The incidence of cancer in the oral cavity can vary based on multiple factors, including geographical location, population demographics, lifestyle choices, and access to healthcare.

Oral cavity cancer refers to malignant tumors that arise in various structures within the oral cavity, such as the lips, tongue, gingiva, floor of the mouth, the lining of the cheeks, and even intraosseous in the jaw bones. It is important to note that the incidence can differ depending on the specific site within the oral cavity [5].

According to global cancer statistics, oral cavity cancer is more common in men than in women. Men tend to have a higher overall incidence of oral cavity cancer, particularly in certain regions of the world. The exact incidence rates can vary significantly between countries and populations. Globally, the incidence of cancer in the oral cavity in men is 1/60, i.e. 1.7%, and in women, the percentage drops to 0.71% [6].

Factors such as tobacco and alcohol use, exposure to certain carcinogens, poor oral hygiene, human papillomavirus (HPV) infection, and dietary habits are known risk factors for oral cavity cancer. Men may have higher rates of tobacco and alcohol consumption, which are significant contributors to the development of oral cavity cancer [6].

> (Tip 3): But who said that we (dentists) conduct a histopathological study to look for cancer existence or assure it is not there only?!

Although oral cancers continue to be the most dreadful lesions, dentists encounter more frequent abnormalities within the oral cavity, necessitating them to ensure accurate diagnoses.

The incidence of ***odontogenic cysts and tumors*** exceeds the rates of cancer. They are common lesions in the jaws, and their accurate and early diagnosis protects the patient from many complications:

1. Not the least of which is reducing the size of the surgical procedure.
2. Material loss.
3. The subsequent relief of subsequent pain.
4. Saving effort and subsequent compensatory cost.

Moreover, an accurate diagnosis and determination of what it is gives an idea about the *possibility of recurrence* and therefore the *time required to follow it up* instead of letting the patient returning after years to lose parts of his jaw.

(Odontogenic cysts and tumors will be covered hereafter through the book).

On the other hand, the diagnosis of **mucosal lesions** is not limited to denying or proving the occurrence of cancer.

A lesion such as ***lichen planus***, which poses a challenge to the doctor and a real problem for the patient, can have its definitive diagnosis by performing a simple biopsy.

Leukoplakia, which is a clinical term, not a histological one, is a potentially malignant lesion, and global statistics say that 5% of clinically diagnosed leukoplakia cases are early-stage squamous cell carcinoma [7].

To repeat the question: why do we need an oral pathologist in everyday practice?

A question that comes to the mind of every dental practitioner, general practitioner, or specialist.

Cases of oral diseases faced by the dentist are usually few, even rather rare compared to a number of dental routine treatments. Still, they might be really quite dangerous; they may need to be referred to a specialist in oral medicine or oral and maxillofacial surgeon and are not followed up by the general dentist himself.

However, this answer, even though it is correct, forgets that the initial diagnosis is the responsibility of the dentist who follows the patient, and in order for there to be a preliminary differential diagnosis, there must be a preliminary knowledge of the clinical and radiological manifestations of the various oral lesions.

For example, most of the intraosseous lesions in the jaws and the most common are:

1. Benign.
2. Silent.
3. Grow slowly.

which leads us to the golden role:

> (Tip 4): Every nonambulatory un-emergency patient must bring a panoramic radiograph to the very first examination appointment.

Oral pathology plays a crucial role in everyday dental practice for several reasons:

1. **Diagnosis of oral diseases:**
   Oral pathologists are specialized in the diagnosis of oral diseases, including oral cancers, precancerous lesions, infections, immune-mediated conditions, and developmental abnormalities. By accurately identifying and classifying these conditions, oral pathologists *assist* dentists in formulating appropriate treatment plans and providing optimal patient care.
2. **Early detection of oral cancer:**
   Oral pathologists play a critical role in the early detection of oral cancers. Regular oral examinations, including screenings for suspicious lesions, allow for the timely identification of potentially malignant or malignant growths. Early detection increases the chances of successful treatment and improved patient outcomes.
3. **Biopsy and histopathological examination:**
   When a suspicious lesion or abnormality is identified, oral pathologists perform histopathological examinations to evaluate the nature of the tissue and provide a definitive diagnosis. Histopathology enables dentists to accurately differentiate between benign and malignant conditions, guiding treatment decisions and determining the extent of surgical intervention.
4. **Treatment planning and prognosis:**
   Oral pathologists provide essential information for treatment planning and prognosis. Their expertise helps dentists understand the behavior and characteristics of oral diseases, including growth patterns, invasiveness, and likelihood of

recurrence. This knowledge influences treatment decisions, such as the extent of surgical excision, the need for adjuvant therapies, and long-term monitoring strategies.

5. **Management of oral manifestations of systemic diseases:**

Many systemic diseases can manifest with oral signs and symptoms. Oral pathologists are skilled in recognizing and diagnosing these manifestations, which may include immune-mediated conditions, infectious diseases, or systemic conditions with oral involvement. Identifying these oral manifestations helps dentists collaborate with medical professionals to manage the underlying systemic conditions effectively.

6. **Collaboration within a multidisciplinary team:**

Oral pathologists often collaborate with other dental and medical specialists as part of a multidisciplinary team. This teamwork ensures comprehensive patient care and coordinated treatment planning. By consulting with oral pathologists, dentists can tap into their expertise, receive second opinions, and benefit from the collective knowledge of the team.

7. **Patient education and counseling:**

Oral pathologists play a role in patient education and counseling regarding oral diseases, treatment options, and prevention strategies. They help patients understand their conditions, potential risks, and the importance of regular oral screenings. Patient education contributes to improved oral health outcomes and proactive disease management.

> (Tip 5): In summary, incorporating oral pathology into everyday dental practice enhances diagnostic accuracy, improves treatment planning, facilitates early detection of oral cancers, and ensures comprehensive patient care.

> (Tip 6): Collaboration with oral pathologists helps dentists provide optimal treatment outcomes, manage oral manifestations of systemic diseases, and educate patients about their oral health.

1.2.2 When to Decide to Perform Biopsy?

The panoramic radiograph may reveal clinically hidden lesions, and an accurate diagnosis can only be determined by subjecting the lesion to microscopic histological examination.

In addition, any lesion that does not respond to treatment must be removed and undergo a microscopic examination to determine the final diagnosis.

This leads us to the next golden role:

1.2 Introductory Guides in Oral Biopsies

(Tip 7): Every tissue removed from the human body must undergo a microscopic study to determine the final diagnosis (Fig. 1.1: the ultimate benefit from biopsy).

The decision to perform a biopsy in dental daily practice is typically based on several factors and clinical judgment. While each case may have unique considerations, here are some common situations in which a biopsy may be warranted:

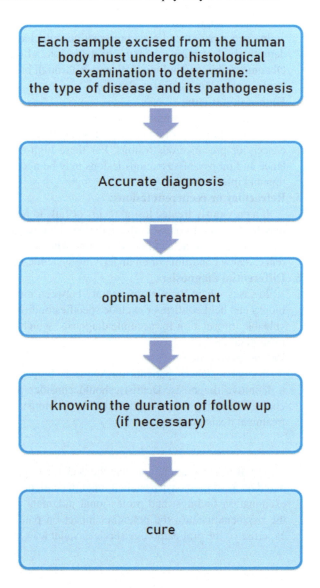

Fig. 1.1 (Benefit of biopsy) Each sample excised from the human body must undergo histological examination to determine: the type of disease and its pathogenesis → accurate diagnosis → optimal treatment → knowing the duration of follow-up (if necessary) → cure

1. **Suspicious oral lesions:**

   Biopsy is recommended when there are suspicious oral lesions that exhibit concerning features such as persistent ulcers, nonhealing wounds, red or white patches, or lumps. Lesions that appear atypical or fail to respond to conservative management should raise suspicion and prompt consideration for biopsy.

2. **Persistent or progressive lesions:**

   If a lesion in the oral cavity persists for an extended period or shows progressive growth despite appropriate treatment and follow-up, a biopsy may be necessary. This is especially important when there is a concern for potentially malignant or malignant conditions.

3. **Uncertain diagnosis:**

   In cases where the clinical presentation is unclear and the dentist is unable to definitively determine the nature of the lesion, a biopsy is often recommended. Obtaining a histopathological diagnosis through biopsy can provide clarity and guide appropriate treatment planning.

4. **High-risk patients:**

   Patients with a history of tobacco or alcohol use, HPV infection, immunosuppression, or previous oral malignances may be at higher risk for developing oral cancers or precancerous lesions. For these high-risk patients, regular surveillance and biopsy of suspicious lesions may be necessary to ensure early detection and intervention.

5. **Refractory or recurrent lesions:**

   If a previously treated lesion recurs or fails to respond to treatment, a biopsy may be required to reassess the pathology and guide further management decisions. Biopsy results can help determine whether the lesion represents a recurrence, a new condition, or an underlying systemic issue.

6. **Differential diagnosis:**

   In cases where there is uncertainty between multiple potential diagnoses, a biopsy can help confirm or exclude specific conditions. Biopsy findings provide valuable information for accurate diagnosis, which influences subsequent treatment planning.

7. **Patient preference:**

   In some instances, patients may request a biopsy for peace of mind or to have a definitive diagnosis. Dentists should consider patient concerns and preferences, discussing the benefits and risks of biopsy and its potential impact on treatment decisions.

(Tip 8): It is important to note that the decision to perform a biopsy should be based on a comprehensive evaluation of the patient's clinical history, physical examination findings, and professional judgment. Dentists should consider the risk/benefit ratio, the potential impact on patient management, and the expertise of the oral pathology service available.

1.2 Introductory Guides in Oral Biopsies

Consultation with an oral and maxillofacial pathologist can provide valuable insights and guidance in determining the need for a biopsy, selecting the appropriate biopsy technique, and interpreting the histopathological results to aid in patient care.

1.2.3 What Types of Biopsies a Dentist Can Perform?

Now that we know that intraosseous lesions and chronic lesions that are refractory to treatment for more than 2 weeks must be surgically intervened to take a biopsy, we must remember the types of biopsies that the dentist can perform [8].

Dentists can perform several types of biopsies, depending on the specific needs of the patient and the nature of the lesion [9].

The most common biopsies in daily dental practice are either **incisional** biopsies or **excisional** biopsies. There is a third type that dentists prefer but oral pathologists do not like, which is FNA (fine needle aspiration) biopsies; other less frequently used types of biopsies still exist in dental practice.

Here are the types of biopsies that can be performed in dental service:

1. ***Incisional Biopsy*** is performed to investigate the lesion by taking ***part of it*** with a healthy adjacent side for comparison; it is useful in *large lesions.*

   This type of biopsy involves removing a portion of the suspicious lesion for examination. It is typically performed when the lesion is large, and complete removal would be impractical or disfiguring. Incisional biopsies provide a representative sample of the lesion for histopathological analysis, allowing for ***accurate diagnosis*** and **appropriate *treatment planning*.**
2. As for the ***Excisional Biopsy***, the ***whole lesion*** is taken at once; to be subjected to microscopic examination; it is usually performed by the dentist for *small lesions.*

   Excisional biopsies involve the complete removal of the entire lesion, along with a margin of healthy tissue. They are usually performed for smaller lesions or when the suspicion of malignancy is low. Excisional biopsies aim to both ***diagnose*** and ***treat*** the lesion as long as it is safe and feasible to do so.
3. ***Punch Biopsy:*** A punch biopsy involves using a circular cutting instrument (a biopsy punch) to remove a ***small cylindrical core*** of tissue from the lesion. It is particularly useful for obtaining ***deep and full-thickness samples*** of the lesion. Punch biopsies are commonly used for lesions with distinct borders or those located in areas with adequate accessibility.
4. ***Brush Biopsy:*** Brush biopsies involve using a specialized brush to collect surface cells from the suspicious lesion. The collected cells are then transferred onto a glass slide for examination. Brush biopsies are minimally invasive and can be useful for ***initial screening*** or when obtaining a conventional tissue biopsy is challenging or not feasible.
5. ***Fine-needle aspiration (FNA) biopsy***: FNA biopsy is a technique that involves inserting a thin needle into a suspicious lesion to aspirate cells or fluid for analysis. This type of biopsy is commonly used for palpable or accessible lesions,

such as cysts or enlarged lymph nodes, to obtain cellular material for cytological examination. FNA biopsies are often performed in collaboration with oral and maxillofacial surgeons or other specialists [2].

The dentist likes a **fine-needle aspiration biopsy** for its convenience. It is performed by inserting a thin needle into the lesion (usually an intraosseous lesion) and aspirating the fluid contained within it (if any), and then this fluid is studied in the histopathological laboratory. It is easy to perform; still, its accuracy is under doubt [10].

Fine needle aspiration (FNA) biopsy of intra-oral lesions primarily serves to communicate one crucial aspect to general practitioners: whether the lesion they are dealing with is cystic in nature. However, its contribution to refining diagnostic accuracy for oral lesions is limited, as the rate of diagnostic certainty for such lesions typically falls within the range of 40–60% [11, 12]. The FNA biopsy provides more of a suspicion level rather than yielding definitive diagnostic percentages in the realm of oral lesions [4].

(Tip 9): Because FNA biopsy is not considered diagnostic in intra-oral lesions, the dentist resorts to surgical biopsy of its two common types (incisional or excisional) and each has its own indications.

1.2.4 Factors Influencing the Type of Biopsy Selection

It is important to note that while dentists can perform certain types of biopsies, the choice of biopsy technique may depend on various factors, including the size, location, and nature of the lesion, as well as the dentist's expertise and available resources. In some cases, dentists may refer patients to oral and maxillofacial surgeons or oral pathologists for more complex or extensive biopsies.

Collaboration with specialists ensures that the most appropriate biopsy technique is employed and that patients receive comprehensive care throughout the diagnostic process.

The most important factor in deciding whether a biopsy should be incisional or excisional (after examining the anatomical neighborhood) is the *size of the lesion.* Small lesions are typically removed in a single session (Fig. 1.2: excisional biopsy), while larger lesions are investigated by sampling a portion to identify its nature (Fig. 1.3: incisional biopsy).

There are many other factors for deciding the type of biopsy (incisional or excisional) that we will go through in a timely manner, but the most dangerous of them is whether the lesion is vascular.

(Tip 10): When the lesion is suspected to be vascular, the intervention must be done by the surgeon and only in the hospital.

1.2 Introductory Guides in Oral Biopsies

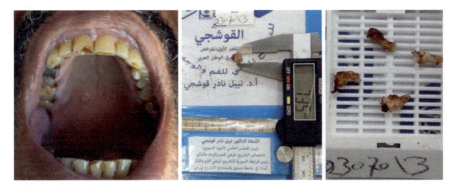

Fig. 1.2 (Excisional biopsy) Small soft tissue lesion in the palate; the decision should be excisional biopsy

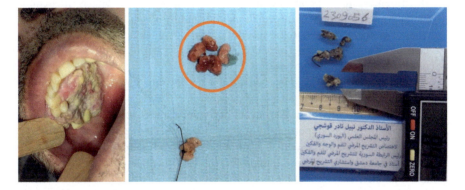

Fig. 1.3 (Incisional biopsy) Large soft tissue lesion in the palate; the decision should be incisional biopsy

1.2.5 How to Handle and Transport Biopsy?

(Tip 11): Proper handling and transportation of biopsies are crucial to ensure the integrity and viability of the tissue sample, as well as accurate histopathological analysis.

Here are some important considerations for handling and transporting biopsies:

1. **Sterile technique**: Use aseptic techniques during the biopsy procedure to minimize the risk of contamination. This includes wearing appropriate personal protective equipment (PPE), such as gloves and using sterile instruments.
2. **Fixation**: After obtaining the biopsy specimen, promptly place it in an appropriate fixative solution. The most commonly used fixative for oral biopsies is 10%

neutral buffered formalin. Ensure that the biopsy specimen is fully immersed in the fixative to preserve the cellular structure and prevent tissue degradation. Follow the recommended fixation time, typically 24–48 h, as per standard protocols.

(The critical role of fixation will be thoroughly addressed in the upcoming pages.)

3. **Labeling**: Accurate and clear labeling is essential for proper specimen identification and tracking. Label the container or vial with the patient's name, unique identifier (e.g., patient ID or medical record number), date and time of the biopsy, and the site or location from which the biopsy was obtained. Use waterproof and indelible markers to prevent label smudging or fading.

4. **Packaging**: Place the biopsy container securely in a leak-proof secondary container, such as a specimen bag or a tightly sealed plastic container. This ensures that any leakage or spills are contained and do not compromise the integrity of other samples or transportation containers.

5. **Documentation**: Maintain detailed documentation of the biopsy procedure, including relevant patient information, clinical history, and any specific instructions or concerns related to the specimen. This documentation assists the receiving laboratory or oral maxillofacial pathologist in providing accurate interpretations and diagnoses.

   (The critical role of documentation will be thoroughly addressed in the upcoming pages.)

6. **Transportation medium**: To prevent drying or damage to the specimen during transportation, it is important to ensure proper packaging. Use an appropriate transportation medium, such as absorbent material or gauze dampened with the fixative solution, to surround and protect the biopsy container within the secondary container.

   (The critical role of transportation medium will be thoroughly addressed in the upcoming pages.)

7. **Temperature control**: Depending on the specific requirements of the fixative solution and transportation regulations, consider using cold packs or refrigeration to maintain an appropriate temperature during transport. However, avoid freezing the biopsy specimens unless specifically instructed to do so.

8. **Prompt delivery**: Arrange for prompt delivery of the biopsy specimen to the designated laboratory or oral pathology service. Minimize delays and consider using reliable and expedited courier services to ensure timely delivery.

It is crucial to adhere to local regulations and guidelines regarding the handling and transportation of biopsies. Specific institutions or laboratories may have additional requirements or preferences for handling and transporting specimens, so it is important to communicate and follow their instructions accordingly.

(Tip 12): By following proper handling and transportation protocols, the biopsy specimen can maintain its integrity, allowing for accurate histopathological analysis and timely diagnosis.

1.2.6 What Is the Fluid with which to Transport the Biopsy to the Pathology Lab?

The most commonly used fluid to transport biopsy specimens to the pathology lab is 10% *neutral buffered formalin (NBF)*. Formalin is a solution containing formaldehyde, which acts as a fixative to preserve the tissue's cellular structure and prevent degradation. The buffering agents in neutral buffered formalin help maintain the pH balance, ensuring optimal fixation of the specimen [13, 14].

Here are some important considerations regarding the use of 10% neutral buffered formalin for transporting biopsy specimens:

1. **Proper concentration:**
    The formalin solution should be prepared at a 10% concentration. This means that 10 parts of formalin are mixed with 90 parts of a buffered solution, typically phosphate buffer. It is essential to use the correct concentration to ensure effective fixation without causing excessive tissue shrinkage or distortion [14].
2. **Sufficient volume:**
    The volume of formalin used should be sufficient to completely submerge the biopsy specimen. This ensures that the tissue is fully immersed in the fixative, allowing for proper fixation and preservation of cellular structures (Fig. 1.4: amount of fixative liquid).

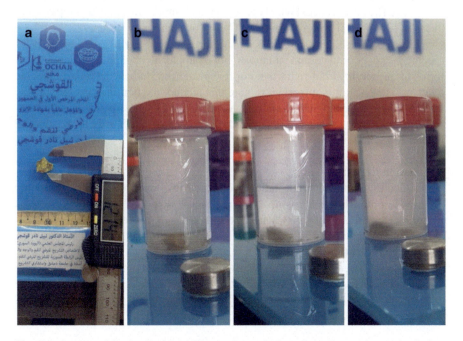

Fig. 1.4 Amount of fixative liquid. (**a**) The specimen. (**b**) Less than adequate immersing in fixative solution. (**c**) Best amount. (**d**) More than enough

3. **Leak-proof container:**

   Place the biopsy specimen in a leak-proof container, such as a screw-cap container or a vial with a tight-sealing lid. This prevents any leakage of the formalin during transportation and ensures the integrity of the specimen.

4. **Secure closure:**

   Ensure that the container is securely closed to prevent accidental opening or spillage during transport. Use parafilm or other sealing materials, if necessary, to provide an extra layer of protection.

It is important to note that specific institutions or laboratories may have their own preferences or guidelines for specimen transport. Therefore, it is advisable to follow the instructions provided by the specific pathology lab or healthcare facility regarding the use of 10% neutral buffered formalin or any alternative solutions for transporting biopsy specimens.

> (Tip 13): The best fluid for biopsy preservation and transfer is formaldehyde. Absolute or even commercial alcohol can be used as a transfer fluid only and not for the preservation of the biopsy.

While ***alcohol*** can be used as a transporting medium for certain types of specimens, it is not commonly used for routine transportation of biopsy specimens in pathology. The preferred and widely accepted medium for transporting biopsy specimens is 10% neutral buffered formalin (NBF), as mentioned earlier.

Alcohol-based solutions, such as ethanol or isopropyl alcohol, can be used for specific purposes or in certain situations. For example, alcohol fixation may be preferred for preserving lipid-rich tissues or for specialized studies that require specific fixatives. However, it is important to note that alcohol fixation may not be suitable for routine histopathological examination and diagnosis.

Here are a few considerations regarding the use of alcohol as a transporting medium in pathology:

1. **Fixation limitations:**

   Alcohol fixation has limitations compared to formalin fixation. It may not provide optimal preservation of cellular morphology and may result in tissue shrinkage and artifact formation, making it less suitable for routine histopathological examination [15].

2. **Specific indications:**

   Alcohol-based fixatives may be used in specific circumstances, such as preserving fatty tissues or for specialized stains or techniques that require alcohol fixation. These situations are typically determined by the specific requirements of the diagnostic or research study [16].

3. **Compatibility with laboratory protocols:**

It is important to consult with the pathology laboratory or a pathologist to ensure that alcohol fixation is acceptable and compatible with their laboratory protocols. Different laboratories may have specific guidelines or preferences regarding the fixatives used for biopsy transportation.

4. **Safety considerations:**

When using alcohol as a transporting medium, appropriate safety precautions should be followed, including ensuring adequate ventilation and proper handling of flammable substances.

It is important to remember that the choice of the appropriate transporting medium may depend on various factors, including the type of specimen, specific diagnostic requirements, and the preferences and protocols of the pathology laboratory. Consulting with the specific laboratory or pathologist involved in the case is recommended to determine the most suitable transporting medium for the particular situation.

To *summarize* the comparison between formalin and alcohol:

It is scientifically known that the best fluid for preserving and transferring biopsy is **commercial formaldehyde** or **formalin**, which is available in hospitals. Academic books recommend the use of a range of preservation fluids as biopsy transfer fluids, but none of them are available in dentists' clinics. While medical references mention that commercial alcohol cannot be relied upon as a preservation liquid for biopsy, it is always available at the dentist's office!

Still, medical alcohol can be a transport fluid for the biopsy, bearing in mind the following:

Formaldehyde has a high *permeability*, which means that it penetrates into the biopsy tissue and fixes it (preserves it) for histological study, while alcohol is less permeable, which means that the (large) biopsy center may be destroyed (underwent necrosis) during transportation, and this problem has a solution.

The solution to solve the permeability problem of commercial alcohol is:

– Transfer the submerged biopsy directly to the histopathology laboratory.
– If we have to delay until the next day, keep it in alcohol in the fridge.
– If the biopsy is quite large, the dentist can help alcohol penetration by making incisions in the sample mass using a surgical scalpel (Fig. 1.5: making incisions in the specimen).

However, please DON'T use saline as a transporting medium under any circumstances!

(Tip 14): The worst liquid to transfer the sample (the biopsy) is the saline serum, and it must be completely dispensed either as a liquid for preservation or transfer.

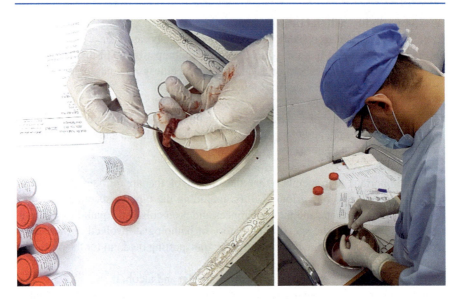

Fig. 1.5 Making incisions in the sample mass using a surgical scalpel

In addition, what about saline?

Saline, or a sterile isotonic solution of sodium chloride, can be used as a transporting medium for certain types of biopsy specimens in pathology. It is commonly used for transporting fresh or delicate specimens that require preservation in a moist environment. While **saline is not a fixative** like formalin, it can help maintain tissue hydration and prevent drying during transportation to the pathology lab.

Here are some considerations regarding the use of saline as a transporting medium in pathology [17]:

1. **Fresh or delicate specimens:**

    Saline is particularly useful for transporting fresh or delicate specimens, such as small biopsies or specimens that require immediate processing. It helps maintain tissue viability and prevents desiccation during transportation.

2. **Short transport duration:**

    Saline is typically suitable for transporting specimens over a short period, such as within a few hours. Prolonged transportation in saline may result in tissue degeneration or autolysis, so it is essential to minimize the transport time when using saline as a medium.

3. **Temperature control:**

    To preserve the integrity of the specimen during transportation, it is important to maintain appropriate temperature control. Keep the specimen container with saline in a cool environment or use cold packs to prevent thermal degradation.

4. **Leak-proof container:**

    Place the biopsy specimen in a leak-proof container, such as a tightly sealed vial or specimen bag, to prevent any leakage or contamination of the saline

1.2 Introductory Guides in Oral Biopsies

during transport. It is important to ensure that the container is securely closed and properly labeled.

5. **Communication with the lab:**

Inform the pathology laboratory about the use of saline as a transporting medium when submitting the specimen. This allows the lab to take appropriate measures and provide specific instructions for handling and processing the specimen upon arrival.

> (Tip 15): Unless a frozen section technique is already scheduled, fresh specimens are not used in routine oral maxillofacial pathology service.

It is important to note that the suitability of saline as a transporting medium may vary depending on the specific specimen type, transportation duration, and the protocols of the pathology laboratory. Consultation with the specific laboratory or pathologist involved in the case is recommended to ensure that saline is an appropriate choice for transporting the biopsy specimen in your specific situation.

> (Tip 16): Again, please do not use saline as a transporting medium for oral biopsies; instead, use alcohol if formalin is not available.

Having described all the main three transporting mediums in dental practice, concluding that saline is the worst, we have to keep in mind that there is one big use for saline in the oral biopsies journey from the dental clinic to the oral pathology service, and it is explained as follows (Fig. 1.6: rinsing the fresh sample):

Once the biopsy has been acquired and prior to its immersion in the transfer medium, it necessitates meticulous cleansing to eliminate any residual traces of blood clots.

It is imperative to bear in mind that the transport medium harbors both preservative and fixative attributes, thereby capable of fixing blood fluids. Consequently, this fixation process has the potential to disrupt the histological depiction, possibly leading to diagnostic inaccuracies. Additionally, the cleansing of the biopsy holds utility in the expulsion of cystic fluids, particularly when the excised lesion demonstrates cystic attributes. To facilitate this procedure, the biopsy is rinsed using physiological saline serum.

> (Tip 17): Don't forget to wash the biopsy with saline before immersing it in the transfer fluid and sending it to the lab.

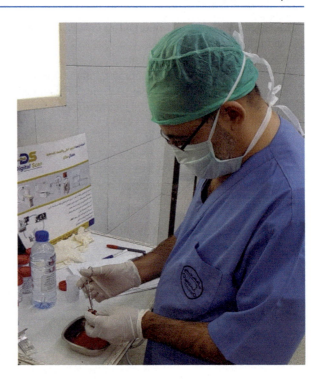

Fig. 1.6 Rinsing the fresh sample in saline

1.2.7 How to Deal with the Oral Pathologist

1.2.7.1 What Should I Write in the Surgical Report Attached to the Biopsy?

Attaching a surgical report with the sample saves a lot of effort and time for the patient and the two doctors (the dentist who performed the biopsy and the "oral maxillofacial" pathologist). Although there is no binding and unified formula for writing the surgical report, there is information that must always be mentioned in the surgical report (Figs. 1.7 and 1.8) and is generally divided into a section related to the patient and a section related to the biopsy itself.

When composing a surgical report that accompanies a biopsy, it is imperative to incorporate crucial details pertaining to both the procedure and the biopsy specimen. While precise prerequisites may exhibit variations, the following are fundamental elements typically encompassed within a surgical report for a biopsy [17]:

1. **Patient information:**
   Begin the report by stating the patient's identifying information, including their full name, age, gender, and any relevant medical record or identification numbers.
2. **Date and location of the procedure:**
   Clearly indicate the date and the specific location where the biopsy was performed, such as the dental clinic or hospital.

1.2 Introductory Guides in Oral Biopsies

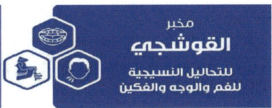

Patient Information:
Name:
Date of Birth:
Gender:
Phone Number:

Lesion Information:
Soft Tissue Lesion:
Color:
Size:
Swelling, Ulceration:
Duration:

Intraosseous Lesion:
Size:
Solid / Cystic?
Radiolucent / Radiopaque / Mixed?
Duration:
X-ray Sort:

Type of Biopsy? Incisional / Excisional.

Biopsy site: please mark on reverse

Transporting Medium?
Lesion History:

Clinical Impression?

Date of Performing the Biopsy:

Doctor Information:
Name: Dr.
Telephone Number: 00963-

Fig. 1.7 The surgical report template. Frontal page: (documentation)

3. **Procedure details:**
   Provide a concise description of the procedure, including the type of biopsy performed (e.g., incisional biopsy, excisional biopsy, punch biopsy), the site or location from which the biopsy was taken, and any relevant clinical information or observations made during the procedure.

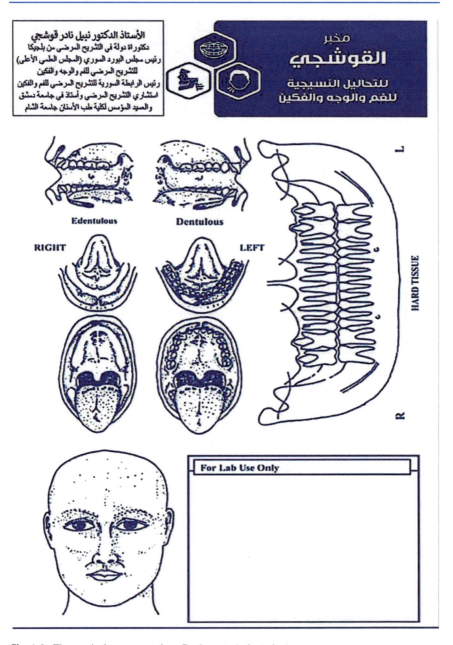

Fig. 1.8 The surgical report template. Back page: (orientation)

4. **Description of the specimen:**

   Provide a detailed description of the biopsy specimen, including its size, color, shape, and any notable macroscopic features. If multiple specimens were obtained, mention them in this section.

1.2 Introductory Guides in Oral Biopsies

5. **Preliminary diagnosis or differential diagnosis:**
   Based on the clinical findings or preliminary assessment, provide a brief description of the initial diagnosis or a list of possible differential diagnoses. This is not the final histopathological diagnosis but can provide important information for initial management decisions.
6. **Specimen handling and transport:**
   Document how the specimen was handled and transported, including the type of fixative used (e.g., 10% neutral buffered formalin) and any special precautions taken to ensure its integrity during transportation to the pathology lab.
7. **Pathology laboratory information:**
   Include the name and contact information of the pathology laboratory to which the biopsy specimen is being sent. This ensures proper identification and communication between the surgical team and the pathology lab.
8. **Relevant clinical history:**
   Provide a brief summary of the patient's relevant clinical history, including any previous biopsies, radiographic findings, or previous treatments. This information can help the pathologist interpret the results in the appropriate clinical context.
9. **Clinician's contact information:**
   Include your contact information as the clinician performing the procedure in case the pathologist needs to communicate with you directly for any further information or clarification.
10. **Signature and date:**
    Sign and date the surgical report to authenticate the information provided and establish a record of the procedure.

> (Tip 18): Remember, the surgical report serves as a crucial communication tool between the clinician and the pathologist. It should be concise and accurate and provide all necessary information to ensure proper evaluation and interpretation of the biopsy specimen.

We will go through each point in detail as follows:

1.2.7.2 Patient Information to Be Included in the Surgical Report

While seemingly fundamental, the inclusion of patient particulars such as name, age, and gender might appear self-evident. However, the significance of articulating these particulars gains prominence when considering instances where physicians draft surgical reports manually or via their personal computing systems, lacking a standardized template for recording information. This underscores the crucial nature of detailing these specifics meticulously.

The surgical report assumes a pivotal role within the patient's medical chronicle, with its relevance transcending not only the current year but potentially spanning decades. Thus, the incorporation of the patient's date of birth, rather than solely their age at the biopsy juncture, stands as paramount. Furthermore, meticulous documentation of the patient's medical history becomes indispensable. This encompasses any precedent occurrence of cancer in any bodily region, as this historical context might wield relevance in the diagnostic context.

1.2.7.3 Biopsy Information to Be Included in the Surgical Report

1. What is the type of biopsy (incisional or excisional), from where exactly was the biopsy taken, what is the transferring medium, what is the history (case history), and what is the clinical impression?
2. If the biopsy is from *soft tissues*, we should consider the following additional points: the *color* of the lesion, its *size*, the *duration* of its presence in the mouth since discovery, and whether it presents as an *ulcer* or a *swelling*.
3. If the biopsy is *intraosseous*, the surgical report should encompass the following details: the *size* of the lesion, its radiographic characteristics (*radiolucent*, *radiopaque*, or *mixed*) on x-rays, and the type of *radiography* employed (e.g., simple x-ray images, computed tomography, magnetic resonance imaging, or other modalities).

The surgical report ends with the date of the operation and the name and method of communication with the referring dentist.

> (Tip 19): Don't forget the clinical impression (differential diagnosis) that prompted you to take the biopsy.

To elucidate the rationale for recording the aforementioned information, I will provide two analogous scenarios:

If a dentist performs a biopsy on a patient's cheek mucosa and another biopsy on the front of the palate in a different patient without informing the oral maxillofacial pathologist the specific locations of the two biopsies or the reasons for the differential diagnosis that led to their performance.

Both pathological reports stated the following histological description: epithelial oral keratinized mucosa or epithelial oral nonkeratinized mucosa. The logical question here is:

- Does the patient suffer from any disease?
- Why didn't the pathologist write a conclusion for the patient's biopsy?

The reason is straightforward: in humans, the mucosal epithelium that lines the inner surface of the cheeks is typically nonkeratinized under normal conditions. When keratinization occurs, there is a high likelihood that we are encountering a potentially malignant lesion, often indicative of leukoplakia.

In addition, the epithelium of the frontal palate is keratinized, and when the keratinization is lost, we have to suspect lesions that may reach the possibility of malignancy.

1.2 Introductory Guides in Oral Biopsies

In both cases, the absence of a final diagnosis results from a lack of initial information about the biopsy itself. This information, which the dentist must document in the surgical report accompanying the biopsy, is crucial.

> (Tip 20): It is imperative to remember that while "leukoplakia" serves as a clinical term, its histological portrayal is most accurately described as exclusively keratinized oral mucosa, which applies to approximately 95% of cases. The remaining 5% deviate from this norm and encompass squamous cell carcinoma.

1.2.8 Gross Pathology (Specimen Macropathology Examination)

Macropathology examination, also known as *gross pathology examination*, refers to the visual inspection and description of a specimen's macroscopic features during the pathological evaluation. It is a fundamental component of diagnostic pathology that involves the examination of the specimen with the naked eye or with the aid of magnifying tools. This examination provides critical insights into the gross appearance of pathological conditions, aiding in the accurate diagnosis, prognosis, and treatment planning of various diseases.

Macropathology Examination Process:

1. **Specimen Reception and Documentation:** Upon receipt of a surgical or autopsy specimen, pathologists meticulously document relevant clinical information, including patient history, specimen source, and surgical procedures performed. Proper labeling and recording ensure an accurate correlation between clinical data and macroscopic findings (Fig. 1.9: checking specimen orientation).
2. **External Examination**: The external examination involves an assessment of the specimen's physical appearance, including size, weight, color, shape, and any external abnormalities. This step is crucial in identifying macroscopic features that may indicate disease, trauma, or congenital anomalies (Figs. 1.10 and 1.11: sample measurements).

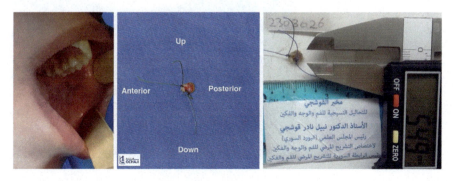

Fig. 1.9 Orienting the biopsy using surgical sutures

Fig. 1.10 Specimen measurement

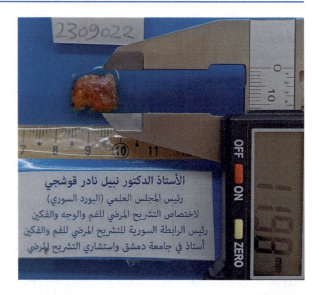

Fig. 1.11 Specimen weight

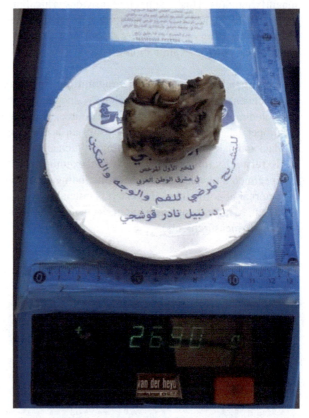

3. **Dissection and Exploration**: After the external examination, pathologists perform a systematic dissection to explore the specimen's internal structures. This involves making strategic incisions to reveal pathological changes and abnormalities within the specimen (Figs. 1.12, 1.13, 1.14, and 1.15: sample sectioning).
4. **Tissue Sampling for Histopathology:** Based on the macroscopic findings, pathologists select representative tissue samples for histopathological examination. These samples are processed, embedded in paraffin, sectioned thinly, and stained to visualize cellular structures under a microscope.
5. **Macroscopic Photography**: Photographs are often taken during the macropathology examination to document the gross appearance of specimens. These images provide a visual record of pathological changes and can be useful for educational purposes, research, and consultations.

Significance of Macropathology Examination:

1. **Accurate Diagnosis:** Macropathology examination plays a pivotal role in identifying gross abnormalities and lesions that may indicate specific diseases or conditions. It guides subsequent histopathological analyses, leading to accurate diagnoses.
2. **Treatment Planning:** Macroscopic findings influence treatment decisions by providing insights into the extent of disease involvement and guiding surgical interventions, radiation therapy, or other treatments.
3. **Prognosis**: Certain macroscopic features can offer prognostic information, such as tumor size, extent of invasion, and presence of metastasis. These factors impact patient outcomes and guide therapeutic strategies.

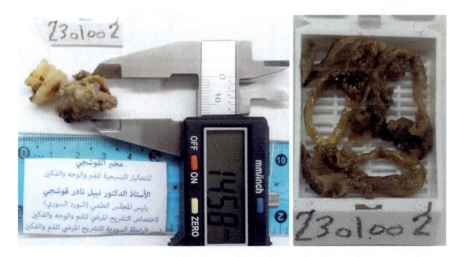

Fig. 1.12 Gross pathology and sample sectioning. When dissecting the lesion attached to the impacted third molar, it was found to be a cystic lesion. Subsequently, histological examination confirmed it to be a unicystic ameloblastoma

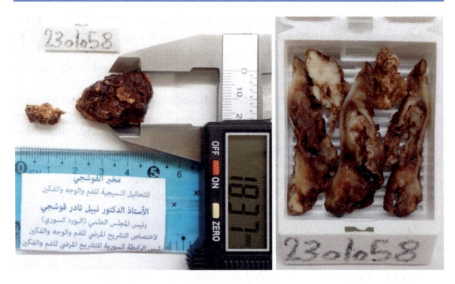

Fig. 1.13 Gross pathology and sample sectioning. In another lesion with a similar clinical impression and radiographic features, the macroscopic examination revealed a solid mass rather than a cystic appearance, the final diagnosis was odontogenic myxoma

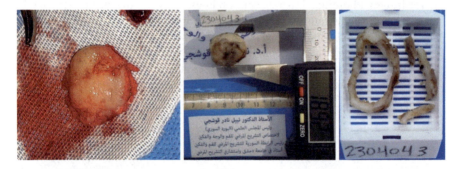

Fig. 1.14 Gross pathology and sample sectioning. Revealing the cystic structure of the lesion

4. **Research and Education:** Macropathology examination contributes to medical research by providing researchers with valuable specimens for further studies. Additionally, macroscopic images and findings are used for educational purposes to train medical students, residents, and other healthcare professionals.

(Tip 21): Macropathology examination forms the foundation of diagnostic pathology, enabling pathologists to uncover macroscopic clues about disease processes.

1.2 Introductory Guides in Oral Biopsies

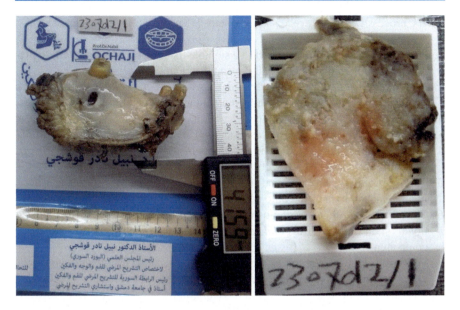

Fig. 1.15 Gross pathology and sample sectioning. Exploring the complete loss of normal maxillary osseous structure and the different coloration of the sectioned area

Macro-pathology observations provide important initial information about the nature and characteristics of a specimen. They help guide further investigations, such as *selecting* appropriate areas for microscopic examination, directing additional testing, and informing the subsequent histopathological interpretation. The macroscopic findings are often documented in the pathological report to provide a comprehensive evaluation of the specimen [4].

This examination is an integral step in the diagnostic workflow, bridging the gap between clinical presentations and microscopic analyses. As medical science continues to advance, the insights gained from macropathology examination remain essential for accurate diagnosis, informed treatment decisions, and improved patient care.

1.2.9 Histological Preparation of a Specimen

Histological preparation is a crucial process in pathology; if conducted by expert hands, half the diagnostic process is already done!

Histological preparation of a specimen is a crucial process in pathology that involves transforming tissue samples into **thin**, **transparent** sections suitable for microscopic examination [9].

> (Tip 22): The goal of histological preparation is to retain the cellular and architectural integrity of the tissue while allowing visualization of cellular structures and pathological changes.

The process typically involves several steps [18]:

1. First, the tissue specimen is **fixed** in a suitable fixative, such as *formalin*, to preserve its cellular components and prevent degradation.
2. After fixation, the tissue is **dehydrated** using a *series of alcohol solutions*, which remove water from the tissue while maintaining its structure.
3. Subsequently, the tissue is infiltrated with a clearing agent, such as *xylene* or other organic solvents, to remove the alcohol and make the tissue **transparent**.
4. Next, the tissue is **embedded** in a support medium, commonly *paraffin wax*, which provides stability for sectioning.
5. Thin **sections**, typically around 4–5 micrometers in thickness, are cut using a *microtome* and transferred onto *glass slides*.
6. The sections are then **stained** using specific dyes or stains, such as the conventional stain *hematoxylin and eosin* (H&E), to highlight different tissue components.
7. Following staining, **coverslips** are applied to the sections using *mounting media* to protect the slides and enable examination under a microscope.

> (Tip 23): The prepared histological slides allow pathologists to study cellular morphology, identify pathological changes, and make accurate diagnoses, aiding in patient management and treatment decisions.

1.2.10 Histological Findings

The purpose of the "Histological Description" paragraph is to provide a thorough and detailed account of the microscopic findings observed by the pathologist. This information aids in arriving at an ***accurate diagnosis*** and ***guides subsequent treatment*** decisions. The description should use precise and standardized terminology, conforming to accepted classification systems and nomenclature specific to the particular pathology or disease being assessed.

Including the histological description in the pathological report ensures that the referring clinician receives a comprehensive understanding of the tissue characteristics and allows for effective communication between the pathologist and the healthcare team.

The "Histological Description" paragraph typically includes the following elements:

1. **Cellular details:**
   This section describes the cellular components observed within the tissue sample. It may include information about different types of cells present, their morphology (size, shape, and appearance), and any specific cellular abnormalities or features of note (Fig. 1.16).

Fig. 1.16 Histological view of radicular cyst. Same case as shown in Fig. 1.14

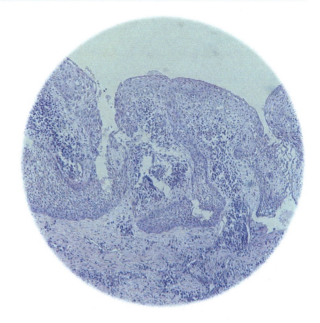

2. **Tissue architecture:**
   The histological description also encompasses the arrangement and organization of the cells within the tissue sample. It provides details about the tissue architecture, such as the presence of normal tissue structures, glandular formations, blood vessels, fibrous stroma, or any disruptions or alterations in the tissue architecture.
3. **Special staining or techniques:**
   If special stains or ancillary techniques were used during the histological examination, such as immunohistochemistry (IHC) or special histochemical stains, this information may be included in the description. It highlights any specific staining patterns or markers that aid in the identification or characterization of the tissue components (Fig. 1.17: H&E vs. IHC).
4. **Specific features or abnormalities:**
   The histological description focuses on identifying and describing any specific features or abnormalities detected within the tissue sample. This may include characteristics such as inflammation, necrosis, metaplasia, dysplasia, cellular atypia, the presence of tumor cells, or other histopathological findings.
5. **Grading or staging (if applicable):**
   If relevant to the specific condition or lesion being evaluated, the histological description may include information about the grade or stage of the disease. This is particularly applicable in cases of malignancies or certain pathological conditions with established grading or staging systems (Fig. 1.18: SCC histological grading).

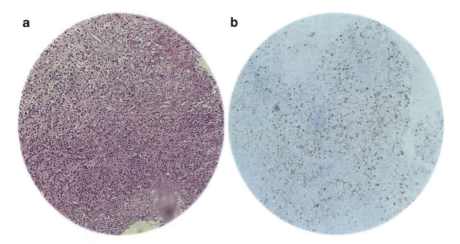

Fig. 1.17 Routine H&E staining, IHC staining. (**a**) Routine H&E staining (left). (**b**) Same histological section with CD20 IHC staining to show B-lymphocytes (right)

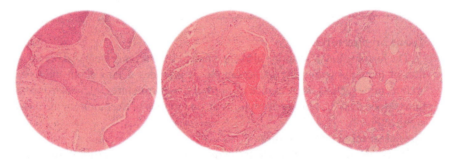

Fig. 1.18 SCC histological grading. Three cases of squamous cell carcinoma, from left to right: well, moderate, and poorly differentiated

To summarize, the histological description part of the pathological report mentions the findings and histological observations on which the final diagnosis is based.

(Tip 24): The histological description often receives insufficient attention within the histopathological report, a facet that is frequently overlooked. Doctors often hasten to reach a conclusion, disregarding the wealth of valuable insights encapsulated within the histological description. It's imperative to acknowledge that this description holds substantial advantages for the effective treatment and ongoing monitoring of the patient.

1.2.10.1 What Is the Importance of Histological Description in Pathological Report?

The histological description in a pathological report plays a vital role in providing detailed information about the microscopic features of the tissue sample. It holds significant importance for several reasons:

1. **Accurate diagnosis:**

   The histological description allows the pathologist to identify and describe the specific cellular and tissue characteristics present in the biopsy specimen. This information is crucial for arriving at an accurate diagnosis. By examining the cellular composition, tissue architecture, and any specific abnormalities or features, the pathologist can differentiate between various disease processes, distinguish benign from malignant conditions, and identify specific histopathological patterns or subtypes.

2. **Treatment planning:**

   The histological description provides essential information for treatment planning. It helps guide the selection of appropriate therapeutic interventions, such as surgery, radiation, chemotherapy, or targeted therapies. For example, the presence of specific biomarkers or cellular characteristics identified through histological examination may determine the suitability of targeted therapies or influence the choice of surgical margins.

3. **Prognostic implications:**

   The histological features observed in the biopsy sample often have prognostic significance. Certain cellular or tissue characteristics can predict the behavior, aggressiveness, or recurrence potential of a disease. The histological description aids in determining the prognosis and potential outcomes for the patient, which influences decisions regarding long-term monitoring, surveillance, or additional treatment modalities.

4. **Research and academic purposes:**

   The histological description contributes to scientific research and academic studies. It provides a detailed record of the tissue characteristics and abnormalities observed, aiding in the understanding of disease processes, the development of new treatment modalities, and the advancement of medical knowledge. Histological descriptions form a valuable resource for future reference and comparative analysis.

5. **Communication between healthcare providers:**

   The histological description serves as a means of communication between the pathologist and the referring clinician or healthcare team. It ensures clear and precise information exchange regarding the microscopic findings, facilitating collaborative decision-making and optimal patient management.

6. **Medico-legal implications:**

   The histological description plays a significant role in legal and insurance contexts. Accurate and comprehensive documentation of the microscopic features provides evidence and supports medical-legal proceedings, including insurance claims, disability assessments, or litigation cases.

Overall, the histological description in a pathological report is of utmost importance as it enables accurate diagnosis, guides treatment decisions, influences prognosis, supports research, and facilitates effective communication among healthcare providers. It is a crucial component of the pathological report that provides essential information for patient care and contributes to advancements in the field of pathology.

1.2.10.2 Examples of Histological Description Importance
There are many examples of the importance of histological description. I will mention some of them and you will find more about them in the next pages of this book.

1. When the diagnosis is **Odontogenic Keratocyst**, the histological description may mention the presence of *daughter cysts* or *epithelial separation*, both of which are indications that this particular case has a high probability of recurrence and needs longer follow-up (Fig. 1.19: OKC histological features).
2. When the diagnosis is **squamous cell carcinoma**, it is very important, given the anatomical peculiarity of the oral cavity, to know the *type of invasion* of malignant cells, whether it is *penetration or pushing*. This information helps the surgeon to estimate the limits of his surgical cut and this information is written in the histological description (Fig. 1.20: patterns of invasion in SCC).
3. When the diagnosis is **periapical granuloma**, noting the *presence of epithelial cells*, *rests of Malassez*, or remnants of Hertwig's epithelial sheath gives the doctor an idea that the condition is a successful endodontic treatment in terms of endodontic treatment, but it remains recurring nonetheless (Fig. 1.21: rests of Malassez).
4. When the diagnosis is **Dentigerous Cyst**), attention should be paid to the following:

   Report the presence or absence of *transformation of epithelial cells* toward ameloblastoma. Approximately, 17% of cases of ameloblastoma arise from neoplastic transformation of dentigerous cyst epithelium.

   Mention the presence or absence of *mucosal cells* in the epithelial lining of the cyst. These cells are a primary suspect in the transformation of the dentigerous cyst into central mucoepidermoid carcinoma (in its early stages, central mucoepidermoid carcinoma resembles a dentigerous cyst radiographicaly) [19] (Fig. 1.22: Dentigerous cyst presence and absence of mucus-secreting cells).

> (Tip 25): When the diagnosis is cystic ameloblastoma, it is necessary to know the shape and location of the neoplastic cells, whether they are mural, luminal, or intraluminal (Fig. 1.23: Ameloblastoma cases).

1.2 Introductory Guides in Oral Biopsies

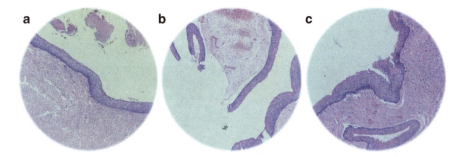

Fig. 1.19 Odontogenic keratocyst histological features. Both cases are OKC. (**a**) (case 1): Without epithelial separation. (**b**) (case 2): With epithelial separation, which increases the probability of recurrence. (**c**) (case 2): Daughter cyst also increases the probability of recurrence

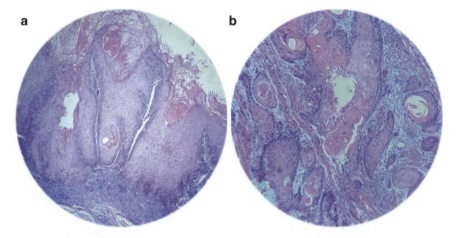

Fig. 1.20 Histological patterns of SCC invasion. Both cases are SCC. (**a**) Invasion pattern is bushing. (**b**): Invasion pattern is penetrating, which increases the probability of recurrence

1.2.11 How Do We Read the Histopathology Report?

Or in other words: What should I (as an oral maxillofacial pathologist) write in a pathological report of a biopsy?

When preparing a pathological report for a biopsy, it should provide comprehensive information about the histopathological findings and diagnosis based on the examination of the biopsy specimen. The pathological biopsy report, just as the surgical report is not limited to a specific form, but in any form it was written in, it must contain the following paragraphs:

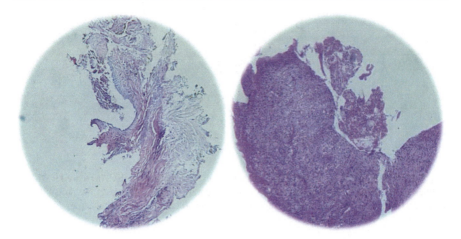

Fig. 1.21 Periapical granuloma cases. To the left presence of rests of Malassez, to the right: absence of rests of Malassez

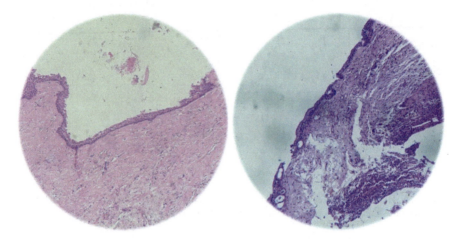

Fig. 1.22 Dentigerous cyst cases. To the left: presence of rests of mucus cells; to the right: absence of mucus cells

1.2.11.1 Patient Information

Begin the report by stating the patient's identifying information, including their full name, age, gender, and any relevant medical record or identification numbers. Also, include the date of the procedure and the specimen accession number or unique identifier.

1.2.11.2 Specimen Description (Gross Pathology)

Provide a detailed description of the biopsy specimen, including its size, weight, color, shape, and any notable macroscopic features observed during gross examination. Include information about the submission of multiple specimens, if applicable.

1.2 Introductory Guides in Oral Biopsies

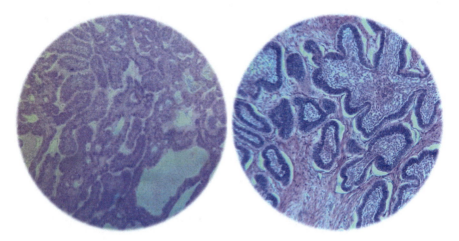

Fig. 1.23 Ameloblastoma cases

If the biopsy is labeled with sutures, it is better to document it with photographs and make the sections go through it as this helps in identifying clear from affected margins.

Some key aspects that are typically observed and documented during macropathology observation include:

1. **Size**: The dimensions of the specimen are noted, including length, width, and thickness. These measurements provide important quantitative information about the size of lesions or abnormalities.
2. **Shape**: The overall shape of the specimen, as well as any irregularities or distinctive configurations, is described. For example, a mass or tumor may have a spherical, irregular, or lobulated shape.
3. **Color**: The color of the specimen is assessed and described. This includes noting any areas of discoloration, pigmentation, or variations in color compared to surrounding tissues.
4. **Consistency and texture**: The consistency and texture of the specimen are evaluated. For example, a lesion or tumor may be described as firm, soft, cystic, necrotic, or fibrotic.
5. **Surface characteristics:** The surface of the specimen is examined for any notable features such as ulceration, hemorrhage, erosion, or necrosis. The presence of nodules, polyps, or other surface abnormalities is also documented.
6. **Margins:** The margins of the specimen are evaluated to determine if they are well-defined or infiltrative. This observation is particularly important for assessing the extent of tumors or lesions and their potential for local invasion.
7. **Surrounding tissues:** The relationship of the specimen to adjacent tissues and structures is considered. Any infiltration, adhesion, or involvement of surrounding tissues is noted.

Moreover, the gross description of the specimen includes:

8. Whether the biopsy is incisional or excisional (according to the surgical report).
9. The location of the biopsy (from the surgical report).
10. Its exact weight and dimensions.
11. Its macroscopic observation while cutting, such as:
    - Metallic feeling upon cutting: lesions as ossifying fibroma might give this impression while doing macropathological examination.
    - Any nodules or cystic structures: cystic lesions with nodules have a higher possibility of having either an acute inflammatory process or a neoplastic transformation.
    - Necrotic center: aggressive rapidly growing malignancies have more likely this phenomenon and it is crucial to document it.

(Tip 26): Expert macro-pathology study is the first step toward a correct diagnosis.

1.2.11.3 Histopathological Findings

Describe the microscopic findings based on the examination of the biopsy specimen. Include details such as the type and characteristics of cells observed, the architecture of the tissue, the presence of inflammation or necrosis, and any other significant features observed. Use appropriate terminology and descriptive language to accurately convey the findings.

1.2.11.4 Diagnosis

Provide the final histopathological diagnosis based on the observed findings. Use standardized diagnostic terminology and classification systems, such as the World Health Organization (WHO) classification for tumors or other relevant classification systems specific to the type of biopsy performed. Clearly state the diagnosis, specifying whether it is benign, malignant, or indicative of a specific disease or condition.

1.2.11.5 Grading or Staging (if Applicable)

If relevant to the specific condition or lesion being diagnosed, provide information about the grade or stage of the disease. Grading and staging systems may vary depending on the specific condition, so refer to established guidelines or protocols for accurate classification.

1.2.11.6 Ancillary Tests (if Performed)

If any additional tests or ancillary studies were conducted on the biopsy specimen, such as special stains, immunohistochemistry, or molecular testing, include the results and their implications for the diagnosis or prognosis. This information provides a comprehensive assessment of the specimen and may aid in further treatment decisions.

1.2.11.7 Clinical Correlation

Discuss the correlation between the histopathological findings and the patient's clinical history, including any relevant clinical observations, radiographic findings, or previous treatments. Comment on the relevance of the findings in the context of the patient's overall condition and any potential implications for management or prognosis.

1.2.11.8 Recommendations or Further Actions

Provide any additional recommendations or suggestions based on the histopathological diagnosis. This may include recommendations for further investigations, follow-up, or specific treatment considerations.

1.2.11.9 Pathologist's Information and Signature

Include the name, professional title, and contact information of the pathologist who conducted the examination and prepared the report. The report should be signed and dated to authenticate the information provided.

Remember, the pathological report serves as a critical document that communicates the findings and diagnosis to the referring clinician. It should be clear and concise and provide all necessary information for appropriate patient management and treatment planning.

> (Tip 27): Every word in the histological report is crucial and should be thoroughly read. Each statement serves as a vital communication between doctors, all in the interest of patient care.

1.2.12 How to Read the Final Result from Pathological Report?

Reading and interpreting a pathological report requires careful attention to the information provided. Here are some steps to guide you in reading and understanding the final result from a pathological report:

1. **Review the patient information:**
   Begin by confirming that the patient's identifying information, such as name, age, and medical record number, matches the individual under evaluation. Ensure that the report corresponds to the correct patient and specimen.
2. **Carefully read the histological description:**
   Although it is far from being a pleasant reading for general practitioners, the importance of reading this section was mentioned earlier.
3. **Understand the diagnosis:**
   Identify the final diagnosis stated in the report. It may be mentioned in the "Diagnosis," "Interpretation," or "Conclusion" section. Pay attention to the specific terminology used to describe the condition or disease. If there are any abbreviations or unfamiliar terms, consult with the pathologist or refer to relevant medical references for clarification.

4. **Evaluate the significance of the diagnosis:**

Consider the implications of the diagnosis. Determine if the condition identified is benign (noncancerous) or malignant (cancerous). Understand the nature of the disease, its potential progression, and any associated risks or prognostic factors mentioned in the report.

5. **Note the grading or staging (if applicable):**

If the report includes information on grading or staging, understand the assigned grade or stage. Grading refers to the assessment of cellular characteristics to determine the aggressiveness or differentiation of a tumor. Staging relates to the extent and spread of a cancerous process. Grading and staging systems vary depending on the specific condition, so familiarize yourself with the relevant classification criteria.

6. **Consider additional information:**

The report may provide additional information beyond the diagnosis. Look for details on specific histological features, such as cellular morphology, tissue architecture, or the presence of specific markers or abnormalities. This information may provide insights into the behavior of the disease, treatment options, or prognosis.

7. **Review comments or recommendations:**

Check if the report includes any comments or recommendations from the pathologist. These comments may suggest further investigations, additional testing, or specific management considerations based on the histological findings. Consider these recommendations in conjunction with the patient's clinical presentation and other relevant factors.

8. **Seek expert consultation if needed:**

If you encounter any difficulties in interpreting the report or require further clarification, consult with the pathologist who prepared the report or seek the input of other healthcare professionals involved in the patient's care. They can provide valuable insights and explanations tailored to the specific case.

Remember, interpreting a pathological report requires integration of the histopathological findings with the patient's clinical history, radiographic findings, and other diagnostic test results. It is important to approach the report in a comprehensive manner and consider all available information to make informed decisions regarding patient management and treatment.

The ultimate outcome lies in the demarcation of the oral and maxillofacial pathology report from the overarching general pathology report. In the forthcoming pages, I will furnish several illustrative examples to elucidate this differentiation.

1.2.12.1 Final Result: First Example

Final Result: First Example (Ameloblastoma)

Ameloblastoma is the most common tumor among odontogenic tumors, and it resembles radiographically many lesions and tumors in the jaws [20].

1.2 Introductory Guides in Oral Biopsies

It may resemble the radiographical appearance (radiologic features) of, for example, *dentigerous cyst*, *primordial cyst*, *odontogenic keratocyst* or *odontogenic myxoma*, and others.

It is an aggressive tumor and tends to recur, but this is not the only problem for this tumor!

(Tip 28): Ameloblastoma is not a single disease. If the pathological report yields only one word—ameloblastoma, it indicates that the oral maxillofacial surgeon is confronted with a significant challenge in planning the surgical intervention.

The following questions will remain unanswered with such a pathological result from the incisional biopsy of an ameloblastoma (Figs. 1.24 and 1.25: the final pathological report):

– How far the surgical margins should be to avoid recurrence?
– What is the best treatment plan?

To confirm, a biopsy pathological report that does not determine the exact pattern of the ameloblastoma in its final result is a tiring report for the surgeon and very tiring later for the patient, unless it is a report of an incisional biopsy and not an excisional one, or the investigation was made by a nonexpert!

Histological patterns of ameloblastoma include the following:

1. Unicystic ameloblastoma.
2. Follicular ameloblastoma.
3. Plexiform ameloblastoma.
   The above-mentioned three types are some of its benign patterns, and the safety margin distance varies among them [20].
4. Ameloblastic carcinoma.
5. Malignant (metastasizing) ameloblastoma.

The last two patterns are the nonbenign patterns and their treatment is completely different from benign patterns [21].

(Tip 29): For all of that, a pathological report of ameloblastoma without determining the exact type is not accepted.

We will continue explaining extensively about ameloblastoma later on when reaching Chap. 4 of this book.

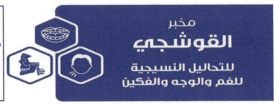

Referring Doctor: *********
Patient Name: Dr.********
Date of Surgical Intervention: 25/12/2022
Date of Pathological report: 05/01/2023
Specimen No. : 2212045

Recurrent uniocular radiolucent lesion in the left mandibular third molar area, the lesion was previously diagnosed as (Ameloblastoma). The surgical sample was a hemiectomy mandible measured in biggest dimensions: 60X34.5X25mm. upon cutting and macroscopic examination the lesion was solid with macro-cystic spaces.

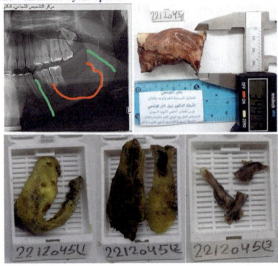

Micro pathology description:

The main showed complete replacement of normal osseous structure with a thick connective tissue that contained islands of odontogenic cells nests (figure 1), these nests jad a plirized columnar peripheral cells and the center ranged between stellate cells and cystic spaces (figure 2). By serial sectioning an odontogenic cystic lining wsa detected, it is the traces of previous dentigerous cyst in the area that had an ameloblastic transformation (figure 3).

Surgical osseous margins were completely free of neoplastic and odontogenic cells (figures 4 + 5).

No atypia nor malignant activity is detected.

Fig. 1.24 First page of the pathological report of a case of ameloblastoma. Unfortunately, the patient himself is a 23-year-old dentist!

1.2 Introductory Guides in Oral Biopsies

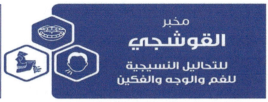

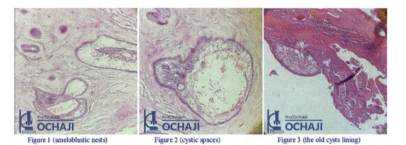

Figure 1 (ameloblastic nests)   Figure 2 (cystic spaces)   Figure 3 (the old cysts lining)

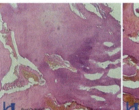 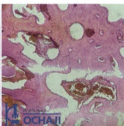

Figure 4 (distal osseous margins)   Figure 5 (mesial osseous margins)

Conclusion:

The surgical biopsy represents: **Mural Cystic Ameloblastoma, with free surgical margins, neoplastic cells were at least 8 mm away from surgical margins.**

Prof. Dr. Nabil Kochaji

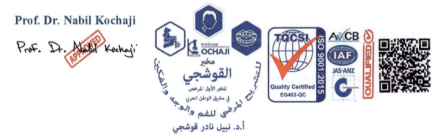

Fig. 1.25 Second page of the same pathological report of Fig. 1.24. It shows the exact subtype of ameloblastoma

1.2.12.2 Final Result: Second Example

Final Result: Second Example (Chondrosarcoma)

The jaws are unique bones in the skeleton from several aspects; one impactful example is chondroma. Chondroma, along with chondrosarcoma and its subtypes (low and high grade), can affect the human skeleton.

However, in the jaws, only low-grade chondrosaroma develops; this is a result mastered by the oral maxillofacial pathologist.

Chondrosarcoma is a rare malignant tumor that arises from cartilaginous tissue. While it most commonly occurs in the long bones and pelvis, it can also manifest in the jaws, although jaw chondrosarcomas are considered extremely rare. These tumors typically present in adults and tend to affect the mandible more frequently than the maxilla. Jaw chondrosarcomas often exhibit slow growth and may remain asymptomatic until they reach a considerable size.

Clinical features may include facial swelling, pain, loose teeth, and difficulty in opening the mouth. Radiographically, chondrosarcomas in the jaws appear as well-defined radiolucent or mixed radiolucent-radiopaque lesions with irregular borders. Histologically, chondrosarcomas are characterized by the proliferation of malignant cartilage-forming cells with varying degrees of cellular atypia and matrix production.

Surgical resection with adequate margins is the primary treatment modality, and adjuvant radiation therapy may be considered in cases with high-grade tumors or incomplete resection.

Due to the locally aggressive nature and potential for metastasis, long-term follow-up is essential to monitor for recurrence or distant spread. The prognosis for jaw chondrosarcomas depends on factors such as tumor grade, extent of invasion, and presence of metastasis.

A multidisciplinary approach involving oral and maxillofacial surgeons, pathologists, and oncologists is crucial for optimal management and patient outcomes in cases of jaw chondrosarcoma [21].

(Tip 30): Low grade chondrosaroma is rare in the jaws, still chondroma is far less frequent!

1.2.12.3 Final Result: Third Example

Final Result: Third Example (Ossifying Fibroma)

Among things that jaws and their lesions are unique is the presence of a ossifying tumor that's subtyped in many ways.

1. Ossifying fibroma (conventional, or not specified).
2. The juvenile variants.
3. Ossifying fibroma trabecular variant.
4. Ossifying fibroma psammomatoid.

1.2 Introductory Guides in Oral Biopsies

Ossifying fibroma is a benign fibro-osseous tumor that can occur in the jaws. It primarily affects the mandible, although it can also be found in the maxilla. Ossifying fibroma is characterized by the replacement of normal bone with fibrous tissue and the formation of immature bone trabeculae. This tumor typically presents in young adults, with a slight predilection for females.

Clinically, patients may experience facial asymmetry, swelling, pain, or tooth displacement. Radiographically, ossifying fibromas appear as well-defined, radiolucent or mixed radiolucent-radiopaque lesions with a variable amount of calcifications or opacities. Histologically, they are composed of a fibrous stroma containing islands or trabeculae of woven bone. Ossifying fibromas can be further classified as central or peripheral, based on their location within the jaws [8].

Treatment usually involves surgical excision with complete removal of the tumor. Recurrence rates for ossifying fibromas are generally low, but long-term follow-up is recommended to monitor for any signs of recurrence. Overall, ossifying fibroma is a relatively rare tumor of the jaws that requires appropriate diagnosis and management for optimal patient care [21].

> (Tip 31): The juvenile variants are different by prognosis and treatment from the traditional pattern, for that a nonspecific result in the pathological report is incomplete result and useless in most of time.

1.2.12.4 Final Result: The Fourth Example

Final Result: The Fourth Example Is Odontogenic Cysts

It is well known that the real cysts, which are the most common lesions in the jaws, are classified as odontogenic cysts and nonodontogenic cysts.

Odontogenic cysts are classified as developmental and inflammatory cysts, which vary with the probability of recurrence, and therefore follow-up period and sometimes treatment.

The developmental cysts has a potential ability to neoplastic transformation to a benign or malignant tumor while there is no single reported case of this phenomena in inflammatory odontogenic cysts [21].

> (Tip 32): Therefore, when providing the final diagnosis, it is essential to draw attention to specifying the exact type of cyst resulting from a jaw cyst. Merely categorizing it as a "jaw cyst" is neither acceptable nor useful.

The worst result is one that does not distinguish between an inflammatory cyst and an inflamed cyst.

To summarize:

> (Tip 33): Final result is the main goal of the pathological study, and it should be as clear and as specific as possible.

1.2.13 How to Benefit from Recommendations Section

It is the top of the pyramid for the benefit of a dentist who treats the patient and the oral maxillofacial pathologist.

The patient thinks, fears the worst, and will look for a word to panic him from intimidating medical terms (node, thickness, invasion of phagocytes, etc.).

The "Recommendations" section in an oral maxillofacial pathology report provides guidance and **suggestions** regarding the *management* and *follow-up* of the patient based on the histopathological findings. These recommendations are typically made by the pathologist and serve to assist the referring clinician in determining the appropriate course of action. The specific recommendations may vary depending on the nature of the lesion or condition identified in the report. Here are some common types of recommendations that may be included:

1. **Treatment recommendations:**
   This may involve suggesting specific treatment modalities or interventions based on the histopathological diagnosis. For example, recommendations could include surgical excision, radiation therapy, chemotherapy, or referral to a specialist for further management.
2. **Follow-up and monitoring:**
   The pathologist may provide guidelines for follow-up visits or monitoring based on the specific diagnosis. This could include recommendations for regular clinical examinations, radiographic assessments, or specific laboratory tests to assess the response to treatment or detect any signs of recurrence or progression.
3. **Additional investigations:**
   In certain cases, the report may recommend further investigations to obtain additional information or to confirm the diagnosis. This could involve additional imaging studies, laboratory tests, or referral for genetic or molecular testing.
4. **Referral to other specialists:**
   If the pathology report suggests the need for specialized care or the involvement of other healthcare professionals, such as an oncologist, oral and maxillofacial surgeon, or periodontist, the report may include a recommendation for a referral to the appropriate specialist.
5. **Patient education:**
   The recommendations may also include guidance for patient education and counseling. This could involve providing information about the condition, its implications, treatment options, potential risks and benefits, and lifestyle modifications or self-care practices that may be beneficial.

It is important to note that the recommendations provided in the oral pathology report are meant to serve as general guidelines, and the final treatment plan should be tailored to the specific needs and circumstances of the individual patient. The referring clinician should consider these recommendations in conjunction with their own clinical judgment and expertise to develop an appropriate management plan for

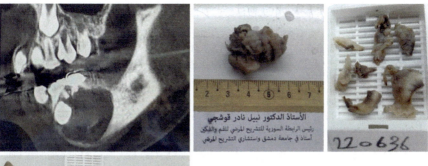
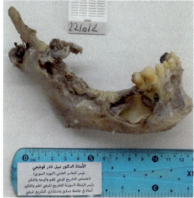

Fig. 1.26 Two cases of odontogenic keratocyst. The first (upper) was treated in a manner time; the second (down) suffered from four recurrences and ended in semi-mandibular ectomy!

the patient. Regular communication and collaboration between the oral maxillofacial pathologist and the clinician are essential to ensure optimal patient care.

To end this chapter of this book, please look at these two cases; it is far different between these two specimens although they have identical the same final diagnosis (Fig. 1.26).

The only difference between each of them is time of surgical intervention and the catastrophe is obvious!

References

1. Dorland WAN. Dorland's illustrated medical dictionary. WB Saunders; 1925.
2. Kumar V, Abbas AK, Aster JC, Deyrup AT. Robbins & Kumar Basic Pathology, E-book: Robbins & Kumar Basic Pathology, E-book. Elsevier Health Sciences; 2022.
3. Miller DC, Karcher DS, Kaul K. The crisis in the pathology subspecialty fellowship application process: historical background and setting the stage. Acad Pathol. 2022;9(1):100030.
4. Farah C, Balasubramaniam R, McCullough MJ. Contemporary oral medicine. Springer; 2019.
5. Farhood Z, Simpson M, Ward GM, Walker RJ, Osazuwa-Peters N. Does anatomic subsite influence oral cavity cancer mortality? A SEER database analysis. The Laryngoscope. 2019;129(6):1400–6.

6. Chhikara BS, Parang K. Global cancer statistics 2022: the trends projection analysis. Chem Biol Lett. 2023;10(1):451.
7. Zhang C, Li B, Zeng X, Hu X, Hua H. The global prevalence of oral leukoplakia: a systematic review and meta-analysis from 1996 to 2022. BMC Oral Health. 2023;23(1):1–15.
8. Regezi JA, Sciubba J, Jordan RC. Oral pathology: clinical pathologic correlations. Elsevier Health Sciences; 2016.
9. Neville BW, Damm DD, Allen CM, Chi AC. Oral and maxillofacial pathology-E-book. Elsevier Health Sciences; 2023.
10. Schmidt RL, Hall BJ, Wilson AR, Layfield LJ. A systematic review and meta-analysis of the diagnostic accuracy of fine-needle aspiration cytology for parotid gland lesions. Am J Clin Pathol. 2011;136(1):45–59.
11. Pons Vicente O, Almendros Marqués N, Berini Aytés L, Gay Escoda C. Minor salivary gland tumors: a clinicopathological study of 18 cases. 2008.
12. Jansisyanont P, Blanchaert R Jr, Ord RA. Intraoral minor salivary gland neoplasm: a single institution experience of 80 cases. Int J Oral Maxillofac Surg. 2002;31(3):257–61.
13. Sheehan D, Hrapchak B. In: Mosby CV, editor. Theory and practice of histotechnology. 2nd ed. St Louis, MO: The CV Mosby Company; 1980.
14. Heslinga F, Deierkauf F. The action of formaldehyde solutions on human brain lipids. 1962.
15. Hammer N, Löffler S, Bechmann I, Steinke H, Hädrich C, Feja C. Comparison of modified Thiel embalming and ethanol-glycerin fixation in an anatomy environment: potentials and limitations of two complementary techniques. Anat Sci Educ. 2015;8(1):74–85.
16. Cinti S, Zingaretti MC, Cancello R, Ceresi E, Ferrara P. Morphologic techniques for the study of brown adipose tissue and white adipose tissue. Adipose Tissue Protocols 2001; 21–51.
17. Lott R, Tunnicliffe J, Sheppard E, Santiago J, Hladik C, Nasim M, et al. Practical guide to specimen handling in surgical pathology. College of American Pathologists 2015:1–52.
18. Bancroft JD, Gamble M. Theory and practice of histological techniques. Elsevier Health Sciences; 2008.
19. Kochaji N. Odontogenic cysts: clinical complications and possible tumour transformation. Brussels, Belgium: VUB; 2005.
20. Cawson RA, Odell EW. Cawson's essentials of Oral pathology and Oral medicine E-book: Arabic bilingual edition. Elsevier Health Sciences; 2014.
21. El-Naggar AK, Chan JKC, Grandis JR, Takata T, Slootweg PJ. WHO Classification of Head and Neck Tumours: International Agency for Research on Cancer; 2017.

Intraosseous Lesions

2

2.1 General Algorism

Creating a comprehensive scientific algorithm for the diagnosis of intraosseous jaw lesions requires a detailed and structured approach. Such an algorithm would involve several steps, considering different aspects of patient evaluation, radiographic analysis, clinical examination, and ancillary investigations.

Below is a scientific algorithm for the diagnosis of intraosseous jaw lesions:

Scientific Algorithm for Intraosseous Jaw Lesions Diagnosis:

Step 1: Obtain Comprehensive Patient History

1. Gather detailed medical and dental history, including past medical conditions, medications, and habits (smoking, alcohol use, etc.).
2. Identify any history of trauma, localized jaw pain, swelling, or other relevant symptoms.

Step 2: Clinical Examination

1. Perform a thorough extraoral and intraoral examination to assess the presence of any palpable masses, facial asymmetry, or soft tissue abnormalities.
2. Check for tenderness, erythema, and regional lymphadenopathy.

Step 3: Radiographic Analysis

1. Review the panoramic radiograph and/or cone-beam computed tomography (CBCT) to identify the presence of intraosseous jaw lesions.
2. Note the location, size, margins, internal structure, and relation to adjacent structures of the lesion.

© The Author(s), under exclusive license to Springer Nature Switzerland AG 2024
N. Kochaji, *Clinical Oral Pathology*,
https://doi.org/10.1007/978-3-031-53755-4_2

Step 4: Categorize Radiographic Features

Group lesions based on their radiographic characteristics [1]:

1. Radiolucent lesions
   (a) Unilocular radiolucent lesion
   (b) Multilocular radiolucent lesion
2. Radiopaque lesions
3. Mixed radiolucent/radiopaque lesions

Step 5: Differential Diagnosis—Radiolucent Lesions

1. Consider common radiolucent lesions:
   (a) Odontogenic cysts (e.g., dentigerous cyst, radicular cyst, odontogenic keratocyst)
   (b) Nonodontogenic cysts (e.g., nasopalatine duct cyst)
   (c) Benign tumors (e.g., ameloblastoma, central giant cell granuloma, cherubism)
   (d) Malignant tumors (e.g., primary intraosseous squamous cell carcinoma, metastatic tumors)
2. Look for margins and borders (well defined, poorly defined borders) [2]

Step 6: Differential Diagnosis—Radiopaque Lesions

1. Consider common radiopaque lesions:
   (a) Benign tumors (e.g., osteoma, cementoma, osteoblastoma)
   (b) Reactive lesions (e.g., periapical cemental dysplasia, condensing osteomyelitis)
   (c) Fibro-osseous lesions (e.g., fibrous dysplasia, ossifying fibroma)
   (d) Malignant tumors (e.g., osteosarcoma)
2. Look for margins and borders (well defined, poorly defined borders) [2]

Step 7: Differential Diagnosis—Mixed Radiolucent/Radiopaque Lesions

1. Consider common mixed lesions:
   (a) Odontomas (complex and compound)
   (b) Cemento-ossifying fibromas
   (c) Adenomatoid odontogenic tumors
   (d) Calcifying epithelial odontogenic tumors (Pindborg tumors)
2. Look for margins and borders (well defined, poorly defined borders) [2]

Step 8: Ancillary Investigations

1. If necessary, perform fine-needle aspiration (to confirm cystic lesions or role it up) or incisional biopsy for histopathological examination to confirm the initial differential diagnosis.

2. Consider additional imaging, such as contrast-enhanced MRI, to evaluate soft tissue involvement and extent of lesions.

Step 9: Histopathological Examination

Evaluate the biopsy specimen to confirm the diagnosis and determine the nature and behavior of the lesion.

Step 10: Final Diagnosis and Treatment Planning

1. Based on the clinical, radiographic, and histopathological findings, arrive at a definitive diagnosis.
2. Plan the appropriate treatment, which may involve surgical excision, endodontic therapy, or other interventions based on the lesion's nature and extent.

Step 11: Long-Term Follow-up

Regularly monitor the patient post-treatment to assess healing, recurrence, or any potential complications (Figs. 2.1 and 2.2: radiolucent lesion in the left mandible).

> (Tip 1): **Conclusion:** This scientific algorithm provides a systematic approach to diagnose intraosseous jaw lesions. It integrates patient history, clinical examination, radiographic analysis, and histopathological examination to arrive at a precise diagnosis. Early and accurate diagnosis is essential for successful treatment and improved patient outcomes in managing intraosseous jaw lesions.

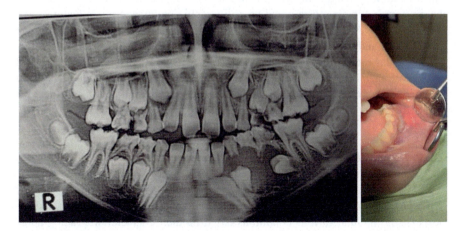

Fig. 2.1 Radiolucent lesion in the left mandibular body causing clinical swelling, attached to nonvital primary molars, and containing impacted premolars

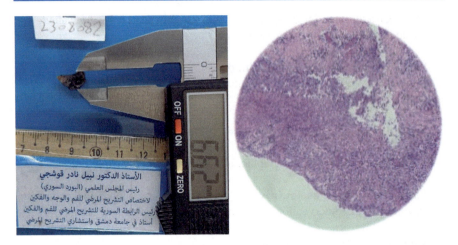

Fig. 2.2 Macro and micro view for the case shown in Fig. 2.1. It turned out to be a radicular cyst

2.2 Differential Diagnosis of a Unilocular Radiolucent Lesion in the Jaws (Algorithm of Logic Thinking)

2.2.1 Introduction

Unilocular radiolucent lesions in the jaws present a diagnostic challenge due to their diverse etiologies and overlapping radiographic appearances. This paragraph clarify an algorithm of logical thinking to aid in the differential diagnosis of such lesions. The algorithm systematically guides clinicians through a series of steps to arrive at the most probable diagnosis based on radiographic findings, clinical features, and patient history. Accurate identification of these lesions is crucial for appropriate management and improved patient outcomes [2].

Unilocular radiolucent lesions in the jaws are commonly encountered in dental and maxillofacial practice. These lesions appear as well-defined, single-chambered (unilocular) radiolucent areas on radiographs, and their identification is critical for proper diagnosis and treatment planning [3].

2.2.2 Top Differential Diagnosis for Unilocular Radiolucent Lesion

When encountering a unilocular radiolucent lesion in the jaws, the differential diagnosis should include various conditions based on their characteristic radiographic features and clinical presentation. Here are some important considerations:

2.2 Differential Diagnosis of a Unilocular Radiolucent Lesion in the Jaws...

2.2.2.1 Radicular Cyst (Periapical Cyst)

This is *the most common* type of odontogenic cyst. It typically occurs as a result of pulpal inflammation and necrosis, and it appears as a well-defined unilocular radiolucency with a rounded or oval shape at the apex of a nonvital tooth. It is often associated with a history of dental caries or trauma [4].

2.2.2.2 Dentigerous Cyst (Follicular Cyst)

Dentigerous cysts usually form around the crown of an unerupted or impacted tooth and present as a unilocular radiolucency with a well-defined border. The lesion often encapsulates the crown of the tooth and can cause displacement of adjacent structures. Radiographic examination may reveal a clear separation between the cyst and the tooth crown [4].

(Tip 2): While dentigerous cyst by definition is associated with impacted teeth, some cases may show partial impaction only; in these cases, the ideal image of capsulizing the crown may not be very clear.

2.2.2.3 Odontogenic Keratocyst

Formally known as keratocystic odontogenic tumor (KCOT): KCOTs are *locally aggressive odontogenic cyst* that can present as unilocular radiolucent lesions. They often exhibit well-defined borders, but they can also appear scalloped or irregular. KCOTs have a high recurrence rate and are often associated with impacted teeth [4].

2.2.2.4 Ameloblastoma

Ameloblastoma is a *benign but locally aggressive* odontogenic tumor. It can manifest as a unilocular radiolucent lesion with well-defined or multilocular borders. The appearance can vary depending on the subtype (e.g., solid or unicystic). Histopathological examination is crucial for definitive diagnosis [4].

2.2.2.5 Central Giant Cell Granuloma

This benign intraosseous lesion typically presents as a well-defined unilocular radiolucency, often in the anterior region of the jaws. It can exhibit internal septations or trabeculae. Central giant cell granulomas are often associated with expansion and can be locally aggressive [4].

2.2.2.6 Aneurysmal Bone Cyst

Aneurysmal bone cysts are benign vascular lesions that can present as unilocular radiolucent lesions with well-defined or multilocular borders. The borders may exhibit a "blowout" appearance due to cortical expansion or thinning. These lesions are often associated with blood-filled spaces [4].

2.2.2.7 Simple Bone Cyst (Traumatic Bone Cyst)

Simple bone cysts are relatively uncommon and are thought to arise from trauma or developmental factors. They appear as well-defined unilocular radiolucencies. Treatment usually involves surgical intervention if the cyst is symptomatic or causing functional or esthetic concerns [4].

It is important to consider the clinical presentation, patient history, and radiographic findings to arrive at an accurate diagnosis. In complex cases, additional imaging techniques such as cone-beam computed tomography (CBCT) or magnetic resonance imaging (MRI) may provide valuable information.

Biopsy and histopathological examination are often necessary if not mandatory for definitive diagnosis and treatment planning. Consultation with an oral and maxillofacial surgeon or a pathologist is recommended for further evaluation and management of unilocular radiolucent jaw lesions (Figs. 2.3 and 2.4: importance of histological examination).

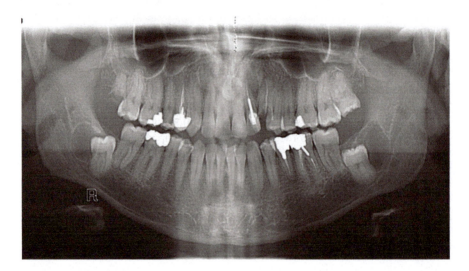

Fig. 2.3 Two symmetric impacted third molars, associated with unilocular radiolucent lesions

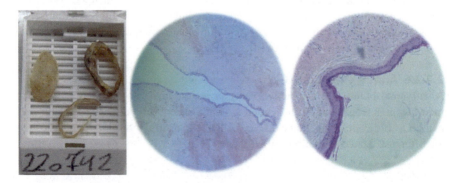

Fig. 2.4 Lesions shown in Fig. 2.3. Both lesions were cystic; still, the right one was dentigerous and the left was odontogenic keratocyst!

2.2.3 Algorithm for Differential Diagnosis

Repeat Steps 1 and 2 in General Algorithm
  Step 3: Categorize Lesion Characteristics
  Group lesions based on their radiographic characteristics: [1].

1. Unilocular radiolucent lesions without radiopaque elements.
2. Unilocular radiolucent lesions with minor radiopaque elements.
3. Unilocular radiolucent lesions with prominent radiopaque elements.

Step 4: Consider Clinical Findings

1. Perform a thorough intraoral and extra oral examination to detect any associated symptoms, such as pain, swelling, or bony expansion.
2. Evaluate the vitality of adjacent teeth and their relationship to the lesion.
3. Check for impaction, partially impaction, tooth missing, and previous extractions in the area.

Step 5: Common Entities for Each Category

1. List the most common lesions associated with each category based on radiographic and clinical findings (write down the most relevant differential diagnosis) [5].
   (a) Unilocular radiolucent lesions with clear well-defined radiopaque borders: dentigerous cyst, radicular cyst, and residual cyst.
   (b) Unilocular radiolucent lesions without clear well-defined radiopaque borders: ameloblastoma, odontogenic keratocyst, and traumatic bone cyst.
   (c) Unilocular radiolucent lesions with prominent radiopaque elements: adenomatoid odontogenic tumor (AOT) and calcifying odontogenic cyst (Gorlin cyst).
2. Keep in mind the existence/missing of tooth, eruption/impaction of tooth, and vitality of related tooth [5].
   (a) *Missing tooth*: Primordial cyst, odontogenic keratocyst, and ameloblastoma.
   (b) *Impacted tooth*: Dentigerous cyst, odontogenic keratocyst, and ameloblastoma.
   (c) *Nonvital tooth*: Periapical granuloma, radicular cyst, and odontogenic keratocyst.

Step 6: Rare Entities and Differential Diagnosis

1. Enumerate less common lesions and entities that may present with unilocular radiolucent appearances in the jaws.
2. Consider systemic conditions that may manifest as jaw lesions.

Step 7: Repeat Steps from 8 to 11 in the General Algorithm

(Tip 3): **Conclusion**: The algorithm of logical thinking presented in this text serves as a valuable tool for clinicians in diagnosing unilocular radiolucent lesions in the jaws. By carefully considering patient history, radiographic findings, clinical features, and auxiliary investigations, dental and maxillofacial professionals can accurately differentiate these lesions and implement appropriate treatment plans for improved patient care. Early and precise diagnosis is essential to ensure timely management and favorable treatment outcomes for patients with uniocular radiolucent lesions in the jaws (Figs. 2.5, 2.6, 2.7, 2.8, 2.9, 2.10: two cases of radiolucency in the jaws).

2.2.4 Vital Teeth

If the unilocular radiolucent lesion is attached to a vital tooth, the diagnostic process becomes even more complex, as the potential impact on the tooth's vitality and function needs to be carefully considered. In such cases, the algorithm of logical thinking should be adapted to incorporate specific factors related to the affected tooth and its adjacent structures (Figs. 2.11, 2.12, 2.13: a radiolucency on a vital molar).

If a unilocular radiolucent lesion is attached to a vital tooth, the differential diagnosis may include the following conditions:

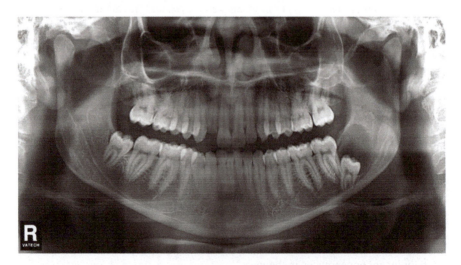

Fig. 2.5 Radiolucent lesion on an impacted third molar. This unilocular radiolucent lesion surrounding the impacted third molar looks like an innocent dentigerous cyst only!

2.2 Differential Diagnosis of a Unilocular Radiolucent Lesion in the Jaws...

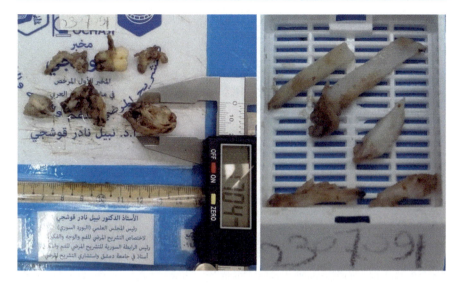

Fig. 2.6 Macroscopic study for the lesion in Fig. 2.5. Macroscopically, it is attached to the neck of the impacted teeth; still, when sectioning, it was solid rather than cystic

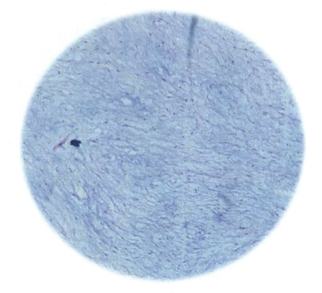

Fig. 2.7 The histopathological view of the lesion in Figs. 2.5 and 2.6. Finally, it turned out to be odontogenic myxoma!

2.2.4.1 Paradental Cyst

Paradental cyst, also known as *buccal bifurcation cyst*, typically occurs around the crown of a partially erupted vital tooth. It presents as a unilocular radiolucency with a well-defined border adjacent to the tooth root. The cyst arises from the periodontal membrane and is often associated with impacted or partially erupted teeth. Surgical removal is usually required [4].

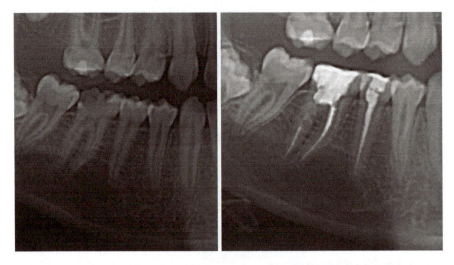

Fig. 2.8 Radiolucent lesion on vital molar. This molar with acute pulpitis symptoms cannot make a radicular cyst; still, the radiolucency exists!

Fig. 2.9 Macroscopic analysis of the lesion in Fig. 2.8. Macroscopic examination showed tiny fragments without specific notable observation

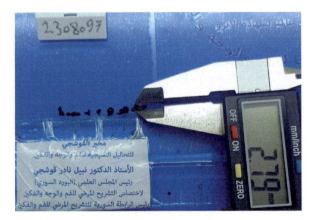

2.2.4.2 Odontogenic Keratocyst (OKC)

Although more commonly associated with impacted or unerupted teeth, OKCs can also be attached to vital teeth. They manifest as well-defined unilocular radiolucencies with a characteristic scalloped or corticated border. OKCs are known for their aggressive behavior and high recurrence rate, necessitating thorough evaluation and appropriate treatment [4].

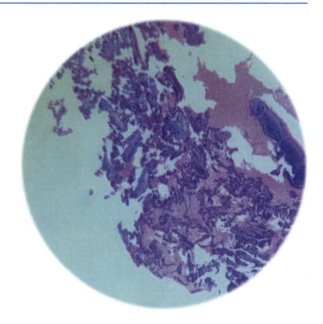

Fig. 2.10 The histopathological view of lesions appeared in Figs. 2.8 and 2.9. Finally, it was proven histologically to be an aneurysmal bone cyst. The case should be before pulp symptoms appear, but there was no radiographic history available with the patient

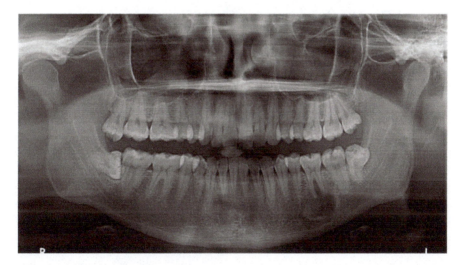

Fig. 2.11 Radiolucency appeared at the apex of the first mandibular molar. The only question mark was that teeth is vital; otherwise, the dentist would call it a radicular cyst only!

2.2.4.3 Calcifying Odontogenic Cyst (COC)
COC is a relatively rare odontogenic cyst that can present as a unilocular radiolucent lesion. It may exhibit areas of calcification within the cystic lining, giving it a mixed radiolucent-radiopaque appearance. Surgical excision is typically recommended [4].

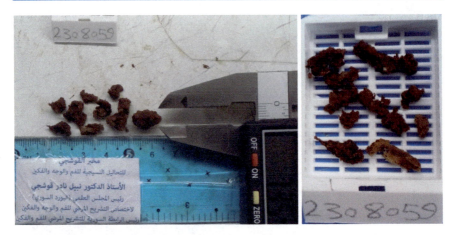

Fig. 2.12 Macroscopic analysis of the lesion in Fig. 2.11. Macroscopically, it was fragmented and could never be enucleated as a one-piece specimen; that was another sign. The third was clear upon sectioning: the metallic feeling!

Fig. 2.13 The histopathological view of the lesion in Figs. 2.11 and 2.12. On histopathological study, the case was diagnosed as ossifying fibroma

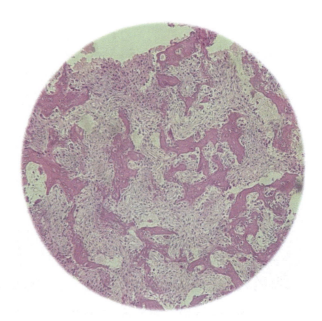

2.2.4.4 Cementoblastoma (Early Stages)

Benign cementoblastoma is a rare odontogenic tumor characterized by the formation of cementum-like material on the root surface of a vital tooth. It presents as a well-defined radiopaque mass attached to the root, often surrounded by a radiolucent halo; still, in early stages, its radiographic appearance is pure radiolucency. Treatment involves surgical extraction of the affected tooth and the associated mass [4].

2.2.4.5 Hyperplastic Dental Follicle

Hyperplastic dental follicle refers to an abnormal proliferation of the dental follicle surrounding the crown of an impacted or unerupted tooth. It appears as a well-defined unilocular radiolucency attached to the tooth. Surgical removal of the impacted tooth and the associated follicular tissue may be necessary [6].

Accurate diagnosis requires a comprehensive evaluation, including clinical examination, radiographic assessment, and possibly histopathological examination through biopsy. Collaboration between an oral and maxillofacial surgeon, endodontist, and pathologist is crucial to establishing an accurate diagnosis and developing an appropriate treatment plan for unilocular radiolucent lesions attached to vital teeth.

> (Tip 4): Conclusion: When dealing with unilocular radiolucent lesions attached to vital teeth, the diagnostic approach should be even more meticulous. By considering the relationship between the lesion and the vital tooth, clinicians can make well-informed decisions about the diagnosis and management, aiming to preserve the tooth's health and function while addressing the underlying pathology. Timely and accurate diagnosis is crucial for ensuring optimal treatment outcomes and maintaining the overall oral health of the patient.

2.2.5 Nonvital Teeth

If the unilocular radiolucent lesion is attached to a nonvital tooth, the diagnostic process still requires careful consideration. In this scenario, the presence of a nonvital tooth may have implications for the differential diagnosis and treatment approach (Figs. 2.14 and 2.15: most common lesion attached to a nonvital tooth).

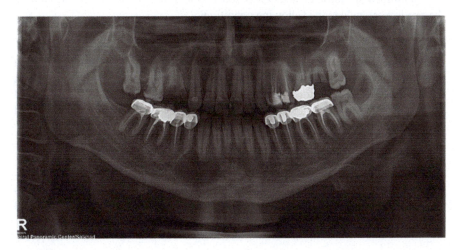

Fig. 2.14 Well-defined unilocular radiolucency at the apex of nonvital canine and poorly treated premolar

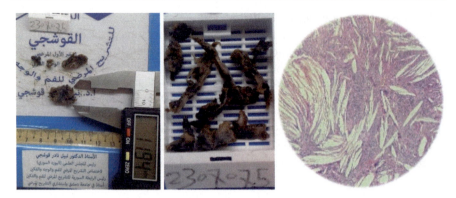

Fig. 2.15 Macroscopic and microscopic analyses of the lesion in Fig. 2.14. Macroscopically, it was proven to be a cystic lesion; microscopically, it was a radicular cyst

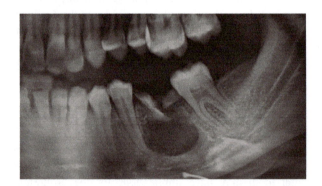

Fig. 2.16 Typical radiographic appearance of a radicular cyst

If a unilocular radiolucent lesion is attached to a nonvital tooth, the differential diagnosis may include the following conditions:

2.2.5.1 Radicular Cyst (Periapical Cyst)
Radicular cysts are the most common type of odontogenic cysts associated with nonvital teeth. They typically appear as well-defined unilocular radiolucencies at the apex of the affected tooth. Root canal treatment or extraction of the nonvital tooth is usually required, along with removal of the cystic tissue [4] (Figs. 2.16 and 2.17: typical radicular cyst).

2.2.5.2 Residual Cyst
Residual cysts can occur when a portion of the radicular cyst remains after incomplete removal during a previous dental procedure. They present as well-defined unilocular radiolucencies associated with the apex of nonvital teeth. Surgical intervention is necessary to remove the remaining cystic tissue [4].

2.2 Differential Diagnosis of a Unilocular Radiolucent Lesion in the Jaws...	63

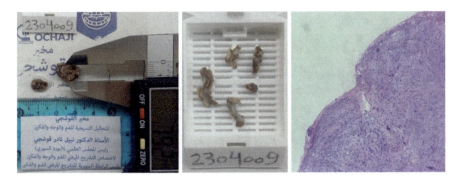

Fig. 2.17 Macroscopic and microscopic analyses of the lesion in Fig. 2.16. Macroscopically, it was proven to be a cystic lesion; microscopically, it was a radicular cyst

2.2.5.3 Odontogenic Keratocyst (OKC)
OKCs can be associated with nonvital teeth, although they are more commonly found with impacted or unerupted teeth. They typically present as well-defined unilocular radiolucencies with a scalloped or corticated border. Surgical excision is the treatment of choice due to their aggressive behavior and high recurrence rate [7].

2.2.5.4 Ameloblastoma
Ameloblastomas are locally aggressive odontogenic tumors that can be associated with nonvital teeth. They manifest as unilocular radiolucencies with well-defined or multilocular borders. Histopathological examination is essential for definitive diagnosis, and treatment often involves surgical resection [8].

2.2.5.5 Central Giant Cell Granuloma
Central giant cell granulomas can occur in association with nonvital teeth. They present as well-defined unilocular radiolucencies, often located in the anterior region of the jaws. The lesions may exhibit internal septations or trabeculae. Treatment involves surgical curettage or resection [9, 10] (Figs. 2.18, 2.19, 2.20: case of CGCG).

2.2.5.6 Ameloblastic Fibroma
Ameloblastic fibromas are benign odontogenic tumors that can be associated with nonvital teeth. They appear as well-defined unilocular radiolucencies, often with mixed radiolucent-radiopaque areas. Surgical excision is typically performed, and long-term follow-up is necessary [11].

2.2.5.7 Calcifying Odontogenic Cyst (COC) (Early Stages)
COCs can also be associated with nonvital teeth. They present as unilocular radiolucencies and may exhibit areas of calcification within the cystic lining. Surgical excision is the recommended treatment [12].

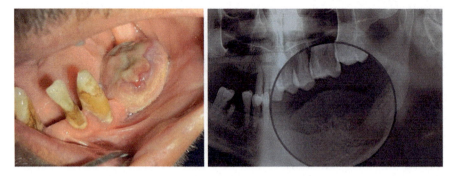

Fig. 2.18 Clinical and radiographic appearance of a case of CGCG. Although peripheral giant cell granuloma is a gingival rather than intraosseous disease, it can make a fingerprint on the underlined jaws

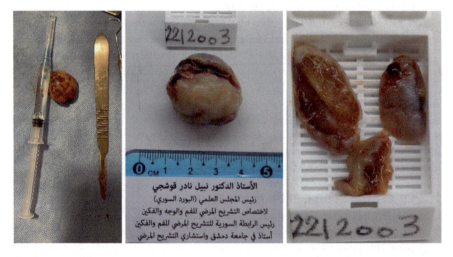

Fig. 2.19 Post-operation specimen. Wide excision to reach the osseous part is essential to minimize recurrence

Accurate diagnosis requires a comprehensive evaluation, including clinical examination, radiographic assessment, and possibly histopathological examination through biopsy. Collaboration between an oral and maxillofacial surgeon, endodontist, and pathologist is crucial to establishing an accurate diagnosis and developing an appropriate treatment plan for unilocular radiolucent lesions attached to nonvital teeth.

2.2 Differential Diagnosis of a Unilocular Radiolucent Lesion in the Jaws...

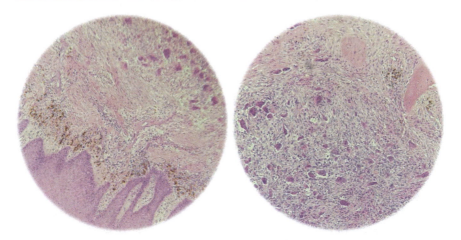

Fig. 2.20 Histopathological view of a case in Figs. 2.18 and 2.19. Just beneath the epithelium, we can see hemosiderin spots due to masticatory forces against the gingiva, and far away the multi-nucleated giant cells are easily seen

> (Tip 5): Conclusion: When dealing with unilocular radiolucent lesions attached to nonvital teeth, the diagnostic approach remains meticulous. Considering the impact on the nonvital tooth and adjacent structures, clinicians can make well-informed decisions about the diagnosis and management, aiming to address the underlying pathology while ensuring the best possible outcome for the patient's oral health and overall well-being. Early and accurate diagnosis is crucial for successful treatment and the preservation of the surrounding dental and maxillofacial structures.

2.2.6 Edentulous Area

If the unilocular radiolucent lesion was located in an edentulous area, the diagnostic approach would need to consider the reason of the absence of teeth and the potential implications for adjacent structures. In such cases, the differential diagnosis may differ from those attached to vital or nonvital teeth.

If a unilocular radiolucent lesion is found in an edentulous area (an area without teeth), all the previously mentioned lesions in paragraphs Sect. 2.2 and beyond are included in the differential diagnosis, except for the radicular cyst. The differential diagnosis may also include the following conditions:

2.2.6.1 Stafne Bone Defect (Stafne Cyst)

Stafne bone defects are developmental defects that occur in the posterior region of the mandible. They appear as well-defined unilocular radiolucencies below the mandibular canal. These defects are typically incidental findings and do not require treatment [9].

2.2.6.2 Simple Bone Cyst (Traumatic Bone Cyst)

Simple bone cysts can develop in edentulous areas and are thought to result from trauma or developmental factors. They appear as well-defined unilocular radiolucencies. Treatment may involve surgical intervention if the cyst is symptomatic or causing functional or esthetic concerns [4].

2.2.6.3 Central Hemangioma

Central hemangiomas are benign vascular lesions that can occur in edentulous areas. They may present as well-defined unilocular radiolucencies. Treatment depends on the size, symptoms, and esthetic concerns associated with the lesion [5, 13].

2.2.6.4 Primary Bone Carcinomas

Although rare, mucoepidermoid carcinoma and squamous cell carcinoma can occur in the jaws and present as unilocular radiolucencies. These lesions require thorough evaluation, including biopsy and histopathological examination, to establish a definitive diagnosis and determine the appropriate treatment approach [9, 14].

2.2.6.5 Metastatic Tumors

In rare instances, metastatic tumors may appear as unilocular radiolucent lesions in edentulous areas. These tumors typically have ill-defined borders and may be associated with a history of primary malignancies in other parts of the body. Biopsy and histopathological examination are crucial for accurate diagnosis and appropriate management [9].

It is important to consider the clinical history, symptoms, and radiographic findings to arrive at an accurate diagnosis. A comprehensive evaluation, including clinical and radiographic examination, along with appropriate diagnostic tests and possibly a biopsy, is necessary for an accurate diagnosis and appropriate management of unilocular radiolucent jaw lesions in edentulous areas. Consultation with an oral and maxillofacial surgeon or a pathologist is recommended for further evaluation and management.

> (Tip 6): Conclusion: When dealing with unilocular radiolucent lesions in edentulous areas, the diagnostic approach should consider the absence of teeth and the potential impact on adjacent structures. By thoroughly evaluating the radiographic and clinical features and considering the differential diagnosis, clinicians can make informed decisions about the management of these lesions, aiming to address the underlying pathology while preserving the integrity of the surrounding dental and maxillofacial structures. Early and precise diagnosis is essential for ensuring optimal treatment outcomes and maintaining the overall oral health of the patient.

2.2.7 Impacted Tooth

If the unilocular radiolucent lesion was attached to an impacted tooth, the diagnostic process would require careful evaluation of the impacted tooth's condition and its relationship with the lesion. The presence of an impacted tooth may influence the differential diagnosis and treatment approach (Figs. 2.21 and 2.22: case of OKC mimicking dentigerous cyst).

The differential diagnosis may include the following conditions:

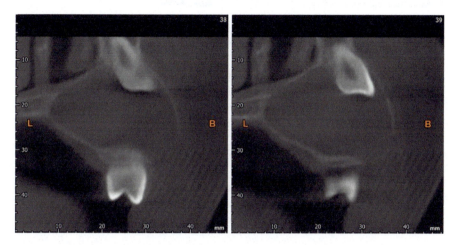

Fig. 2.21 Impacted canine surrounded by a radiolucent unilocular lesion

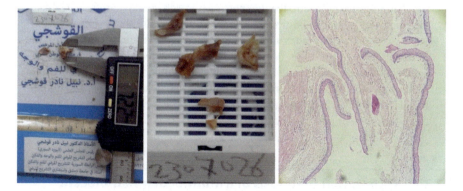

Fig. 2.22 Macroscopic and microscopic analysis of the lesion in Fig. 2.21. Nothing important was visible on macroscopic study, no sectioning clear cystic structure was detected, and histological examination proved OKC case

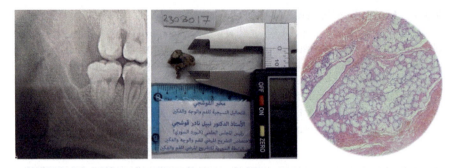

Fig. 2.23 Radiolucent lesion distal of the third mandibular molar. Occasionally in the retromolar area some ectopic minor salivary glands might be detected

2.2.7.1 Top Priority Differential Diagnosis
Top priority differential diagnosis includes dentigerous cyst, odontogenic keratocyst, unicystic ameloblastoma, and odontogenic myxoma [5].

2.2.7.2 Rare Lesions
Rare lesions in the area cannot be ruled out such as the following:
Primary malignancies [5].

Unilocular radiolucent lesions with prominent radiopaque elements: adenomatoid odontogenic tumor (AOT), cementoblastoma (early stages), and complex odontoma (early stages) [5] (Fig. 2.23: rare condition in the retro-molar area).

(Tip 7): Conclusion: When dealing with unilocular radiolucent lesions attached to impacted teeth, the diagnostic approach should carefully evaluate the impacted tooth's condition and its relationship with the lesion. By thoroughly evaluating the radiographic and clinical features and considering the differential diagnosis, clinicians can make informed decisions about the management of these lesions, aiming to address the underlying pathology while preserving the health of the impacted tooth and surrounding dental and maxillofacial structures. Early and accurate diagnosis is crucial for successful treatment and optimal patient outcomes.

2.3 Differential Diagnosis of a Multilocular Radiolucent Lesion in the Jaws (Algorithm of Logic Thinking)

2.3.1 Introduction

Multilocular radiolucent lesions in the jaws pose a diagnostic challenge due to their complex and diverse etiologies. The coming paragraph presents an algorithm of logical thinking to aid in the differential diagnosis of such lesions. The algorithm

2.3 Differential Diagnosis of a Multilocular Radiolucent Lesion in the Jaws...

guides clinicians through a systematic approach, incorporating radiographic findings, clinical features, and patient history to arrive at the most probable diagnosis. Accurate identification of these lesions is essential for appropriate management and improved patient outcomes.

Multilocular radiolucent lesions in the jaws present a significant diagnostic dilemma for dental and maxillofacial practitioners. These lesions appear as well-defined, multi-chambered radiolucent areas on radiographs, often exhibiting a honeycomb or soap bubble appearance. Due to the variety of pathologies associated with this presentation, a systematic approach is crucial for accurate diagnosis [11].

2.3.2 Top Differential Diagnosis for Multilocular Radiolucent Lesion

The coming few lines involve a systematic evaluation of various possible conditions to arrive at an accurate diagnosis. When faced with such a lesion, several pathologic entities need to be considered based on their characteristic radiographic features and clinical presentation (Figs. 2.24 and 2.25: typical multilocular radiolucent lesion).

> (Tip 8): Two common lesions should be excluded when facing multilocular radiolucency in the jaws, namely dentigerous cyst and radicular cyst; although they occupy the top of differential diagnosis in radiolucent lesion, still they are always unilocular [4].

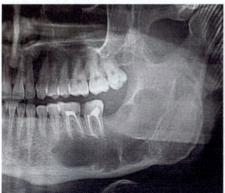 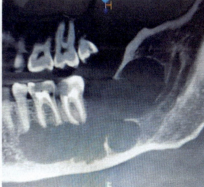

Fig. 2.24 Multilocular radiolucent lesion

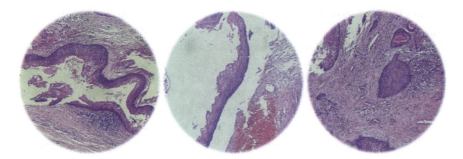

Fig. 2.25 Histological view of the lesion in Fig. 2.24. Histologically, it was proven to be OKC, having all alarms of high recurrence rates, epithelial separation, and daughter cysts

2.3.2.1 Odontogenic Keratocyst
One of the primary considerations is odontogenic keratocyst, which typically manifests as a well-defined, multilocular radiolucency with thin, scalloped borders. Its association with impacted teeth, rapid growth, and potential for recurrence necessitate careful evaluation and management [4].

2.3.2.2 Ameloblastoma
Another potential diagnosis is ameloblastoma, a locally aggressive odontogenic tumor characterized by a multilocular radiolucency with a "soap-bubble" or "honeycomb" appearance. Histopathological examination is often required for definitive diagnosis due to its overlapping features with other lesions.

Furthermore, the possibility of a *unicystic ameloblastoma* should be considered, which presents as a unilocular or multilocular radiolucency with an identifiable cystic lining. This subtype often occurs in younger individuals and may exhibit a less aggressive behavior compared to *conventional ameloblastoma* [4].

2.3.2.3 Central Giant Cell Granuloma
Other potential entities include central giant cell granuloma, which presents as a well-defined, expansile multilocular radiolucency, typically exhibiting aggressive growth patterns and vascularization. The presence of internal septations or trabeculae can help differentiate it from other lesions. Another consideration is an aneurysmal bone cyst, characterized by an eccentric, expansive multilocular radiolucency with a "blowout" appearance, often associated with cortical thinning or expansion [4].

2.3.2.4 Odontogenic Myxoma
One important consideration is the odontogenic myxoma, which is commonly associated with impacted or unerupted teeth. It presents as a well-defined, unilocular, or multilocular radiolucency that might be associated with surrounding the crown of an impacted tooth or in any other area in the jaws. Differentiating it from other lesions, such as odontogenic keratocyst or unicystic ameloblastoma, is crucial due to the differences in treatment and potential for recurrence [4].

2.3.2.5 Less Frequently Encountered Lesions

Less frequently encountered lesions such as ossifying fibroma, central hemangioma, and central giant cell lesion should also be included in the differential diagnosis. Other lesions such as the Pindborg tumor and Gorlin cyst may exhibit varied radiographic features, ranging from well-defined multilocular radiolucencies (early stages) to mixed radiolucent-radiopaque patterns (late stages) [4].

The clinical presentation, patient age, location of the lesion, and associated symptoms should be carefully assessed and correlated with the radiographic findings to reach a definitive diagnosis. In some cases, additional imaging modalities such as cone-beam computed tomography (CBCT) or magnetic resonance imaging (MRI) may be necessary to aid in the diagnostic process (Fig. 2.26: importance of histological examination for every multilocular radiolucent lesion).

2.3.3 Algorithm for Differential Diagnosis

This text aims to provide an algorithm of logical thinking to facilitate a comprehensive differential diagnosis for multilocular radiolucent lesions in the jaws.

Step 1: Repeat Steps 1 and 2
Step 2: Categorize Lesion Characteristics
Group lesions based on their radiographic characteristics: [1].

1. Multilocular radiolucent lesions without radiopaque elements.
2. Multilocular radiolucent lesions with minor radiopaque elements.
3. Multilocular radiolucent lesions with prominent radiopaque elements.

Step 3: Consider Clinical Findings

1. Perform a thorough intraoral and extraoral examination to detect any swelling, erythema, ulceration, or bony expansion related to the lesion.
2. Evaluate the presence of associated symptoms such as pain, sensitivity, or mobility of adjacent teeth.

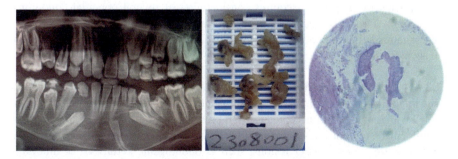

Fig. 2.26 Multilocular radiolucent lesion in the anterior mandible. This huge radiolucent multilocular lesion was thought as a dentigerous cyst, and a marsupialization was scheduled. The incisional biopsy proved it was a cystic lesion

Step 4: Common Entities for Each Category

List the most common lesions associated with each category based on radiographic and clinical findings.

1. Multilocular radiolucent lesions without radiopaque elements: ameloblastoma, odontogenic keratocyst, and odontogenic myxoma [5].
2. Multilocular radiolucent lesions with minor radiopaque elements: central giant cell tumor and ameloblastic fibroma [5].
3. Multilocular radiolucent lesions with prominent radiopaque elements: ossifying fibroma, cementoblastoma, calcifying odontogenic cyst (Gorlin cyst), and calcifying odontogenic tumor (Pindborg tumor) [5].

Step 5: Repeat Steps from 8 to 11

(Tip 9): Ultimately, histopathological examination through biopsy or surgical excision is often required to establish a definitive diagnosis and guide appropriate treatment planning. Collaboration between an oral and maxillofacial surgeon, a pathologist, and a radiologist is crucial to accurately differentiate between these various entities and provide optimal patient care.

2.3.4 Vital Teeth

When dealing with multilocular radiolucent lesions attached to vital teeth, the diagnostic approach should be even more meticulous. By considering the relationship between the lesion and the vital tooth, clinicians can make well-informed decisions about the diagnosis and management, aiming to preserve the tooth's health and function while addressing the underlying pathology. Timely and accurate diagnosis is crucial for ensuring optimal treatment and maintaining the overall oral health of the patient.

Differential diagnosis of a multilocular radiolucent lesion in the jaws, specifically related to vital teeth, requires consideration of several potential conditions (Fig. 2.27). These lesions may arise from various dental and nondental origins, necessitating a thorough evaluation of clinical and radiographic features to establish an accurate diagnosis.

2.3.4.1 Odontogenic Myxoma

One important consideration is the odontogenic myxoma, which is commonly associated with impacted or unerupted teeth. It presents as a well-defined, unilocular, or multilocular radiolucency surrounding the crown of an impacted tooth. Differentiating it from other lesions, such as odontogenic keratocyst or unicystic ameloblastoma, is crucial due to the differences in treatment and potential for recurrence [4].

Fig. 2.27 Glandular odontogenic cyst

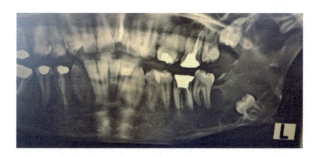

2.3.4.2 Ameloblastoma and Other Related Ameloblastic Family Tumors

Other less common lesions related to vital teeth include odontogenic tumors such as *ameloblastic fibroma* and *ameloblastic fibro-odontoma*. These tumors often present as mixed radiolucent-radiopaque lesions, with the presence of both radiolucent and radiopaque components. Ameloblastic fibro-odontoma may also exhibit an irregularly shaped radiolucency associated with an impacted tooth and dental hard tissue-like structures within the lesion [4].

In some cases, the presence of a multilocular radiolucent lesion associated with a vital tooth may indicate a more aggressive pathology, such as ameloblastoma or central giant cell granuloma. These lesions can present with varied radiographic features, including multilocular radiolucencies with scalloped or soap-bubble appearances. Histopathological examination is essential for definitive diagnosis and treatment planning.

To reach an accurate diagnosis, it is important to consider the clinical presentation, patient history, and radiographic findings. In complex cases, additional imaging techniques such as CBCT or MRI may provide valuable information for a comprehensive evaluation.

A multidisciplinary approach involving an oral and maxillofacial surgeon, endodontist, and oral pathologist is often necessary to establish an accurate diagnosis and develop an appropriate treatment plan for lesions associated with vital teeth.

2.3.5 Nonvital Teeth

When dealing with multilocular radiolucent lesions attached to nonvital teeth, the diagnostic approach remains meticulous. Considering the impact on the nonvital tooth and adjacent structures, clinicians can make well-informed decisions about the diagnosis and management, aiming to address the underlying pathology while preserving the overall health of the affected area. Early and accurate diagnosis is crucial for successful treatment and optimal patient outcomes.

If the associated teeth are nonvital, the differential diagnosis of a multilocular radiolucent lesion in the jaws expands to include conditions that are commonly associated with nonvital teeth. Here are some important considerations:

2.3.5.1 Odontogenic Keratocyst

Odontogenic keratocyst can occur in association with both vital and nonvital teeth. These aggressive lesions typically appear as well-defined, multilocular radiolucencies with thin, scalloped borders. The presence of nonvital teeth can be associated with larger lesions or more extensive involvement [15].

2.3.5.2 Ameloblastoma

Although more commonly associated with vital teeth, ameloblastomas can also occur in relation to nonvital teeth, which might delay the accurate diagnosis and appropriate treatment. Biopsy and histopathological examination are essential for definitive diagnosis [16] (Figs. 2.28 and 2.29).

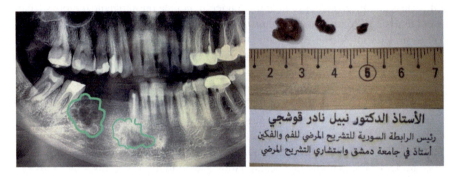

Fig. 2.28 Soup bubble multilocular radiolucent lesion

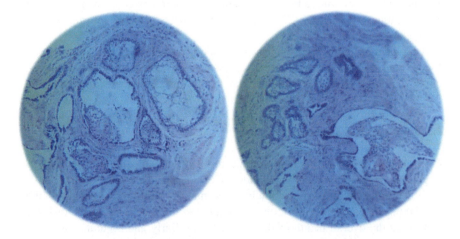

Fig. 2.29 Same case as of Fig. 2.27. The diagnosis is conventional ameloblastoma

2.3.5.3 Less Frequent Lesion

Other less common entities: Lesions such as *central giant cell granuloma* [10] or malignancies like squamous cell carcinoma can also present as multilocular radiolucent lesions associated with nonvital teeth [17].

> (Tip 10): Accurate diagnosis requires a combination of clinical, radiographic, and histopathological evaluation. Cone-beam computed tomography (CBCT) may provide additional information regarding the extent and characteristics of the lesion. Collaboration between an oral and maxillofacial surgeon, endodontist, and pathologist is crucial to reach a definitive diagnosis and develop an appropriate treatment plan for lesions associated with nonvital teeth.

2.3.6 Edentulous Area

When dealing with multilocular radiolucent lesions in edentulous areas, the diagnostic approach should consider the absence of teeth and the potential impact on adjacent structures. By thoroughly evaluating the radiographic and clinical features and considering the differential diagnosis, clinicians can make informed decisions about the management of these lesions, aiming to address the underlying pathology while ensuring the best possible outcome for the patient's oral health and overall well-being. Early and accurate diagnosis is essential for successful treatment and the preservation of the surrounding dental and maxillofacial structures (Figs. 2.30, 2.31, 2.32, 2.33: two cases of tumors that arise in edentulous areas).

If the multilocular radiolucent lesion appears in an edentulous area (an area without teeth), the differential diagnosis may include the following conditions:

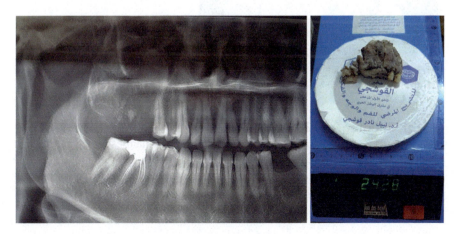

Fig. 2.30 Multilocular radiolucent/mixed lesion in the maxilla. A 2-year delay in diagnosing the case cost this 45-year-old lady the loss of her jaw

Fig. 2.31 The case of Fig. 2.30. It was finally diagnosed as a Pindborg tumor

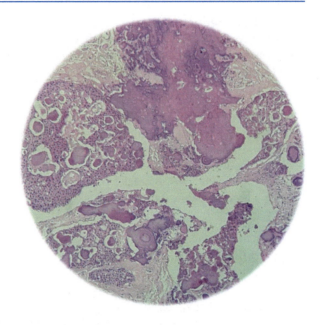

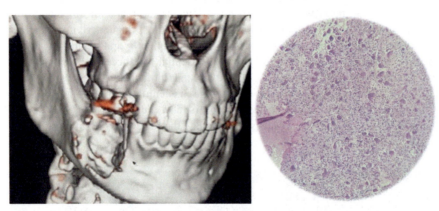

Fig. 2.32 3D and histological view of a sad case. This central giant cell tumor was treated as an abscess for several months!

2.3.6.1 Odontogenic Glandular Cyst

Although it is an aggressive rare odontogenic cyst, its manifestations are still not clear and fully documented. Roughly 200 cases have been reported in the literature and the main problem that exists here is that it can mimic various types of odontogenic cysts and tumors [18, 19].

2.3 Differential Diagnosis of a Multilocular Radiolucent Lesion in the Jaws... 77

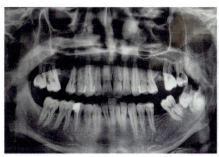 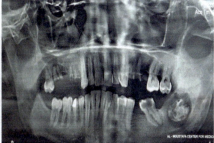

Fig. 2.33 Odontoma development through a 3-year period

2.3.6.2 Central Giant Cell Granuloma

This benign, locally aggressive lesion can manifest in both dentate and edentulous areas. It appears as a well-defined, multilocular radiolucency with internal septations or trabeculae. Treatment depends on the size and aggressiveness of the lesion and may involve surgical curettage or resection [20].

2.3.6.3 Metastatic Lesions

In rare instances, metastatic tumors may appear as radiolucent lesions in edentulous areas. These lesions typically have ill-defined borders and may be associated with a history of primary malignancies in other parts of the body. Biopsy and histopathological examination are crucial for accurate diagnosis [9].

> (Tip 11): Although metastatic lesions in the jaws are quite rare, dentists may save human life by early diagnosis of such cases, especially when the patient is not aware of his primary cancer.

It is important to note that a definitive diagnosis requires histopathological examination through biopsy or surgical excision. Therefore, consultation with an oral and maxillofacial surgeon or a pathologist is recommended for accurate diagnosis and appropriate management of multilocular radiolucent lesions in edentulous areas.

Based on the differential diagnosis and the location in the edentulous area, determine the most appropriate treatment plan. This may involve surgical excision, bone grafting, or other interventions, depending on the specific diagnosis and clinical situation.

2.3.7 Located Near an Impacted Tooth

All the above-mentioned lesions in paragraphs (Sect. 2.3) can appear near the impacted tooth, and the only golden standard diagnostic tool is the histological examination.

When dealing with multilocular radiolucent lesions located near the impacted teeth, the diagnostic approach should carefully evaluate the relationship between the lesion and the impacted tooth. By thoroughly considering radiographic and clinical features and incorporating the impact on adjacent structures, clinicians can make well-informed decisions about the diagnosis and management, aiming to address the underlying pathology while preserving the health of the impacted tooth and surrounding dental and maxillofacial structures. Early and accurate diagnosis is crucial for successful treatment and optimal patient outcomes. But remember, it's definitely not a dentigerous cyst!

2.4 Differential Diagnosis of a Radiopaque Lesion in the Jaws (Algorithm of Logic Thinking)

2.4.1 Introduction

Radiopaque lesions within the jaws refer to areas of increased radiodensity that appear on dental radiographs. These findings, often incidentally discovered during routine dental imaging (normally silent lesions), encompass a wide array of conditions ranging from benign to malignant. The ability to effectively diagnose and differentiate these lesions is of paramount importance in order to guide appropriate treatment decisions. These lesions can originate from various sources, including bone, calcified tissues, and teeth. In the coming paragraph, we delve into the most frequently encountered radiopaque lesions found within the jaws. We will explore their distinct characteristics and discuss the systematic diagnostic algorithm employed to accurately classify and manage these conditions.

2.4.2 Top Common Radiopaque Lesions

Several radiopaque lesions are frequently observed within the jaws, each presenting unique features and considerations.

2.4.2.1 Complex and Compound Odontoma

Odontomas are the most common odontogenic tumors, and they present as well-defined radiopaque masses composed of dental hard tissues.

They can be further classified as complex or compound odontomas based on their structure. Odontomas are usually asymptomatic and are often detected incidentally on radiographs. They are classified as a developmental anomaly and present as irregular radiopaque structures due to disorganized dental tissue growth.

While benign, its potential impact on adjacent structures underscores the importance of accurate diagnosis [4] (Figs. 2.33, 2.34, 2.35).

> (Tip 12): From the wide varieties of oral intraosseous lesions that cannot be diagnosed without histological examination, odontoma is one of the very rare exceptions to this role.

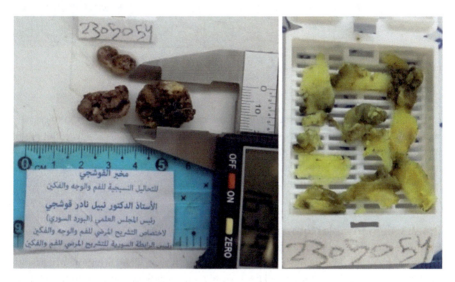

Fig. 2.34 Macroscopic examination of the case of odontoma. Macroscopically, the specimen was very hard; using nitric acid gave the specimen this yellow color

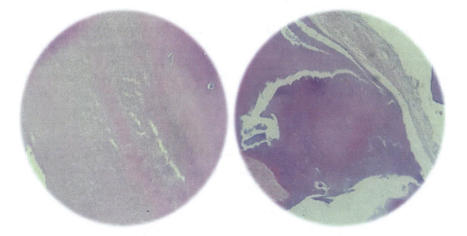

Fig. 2.35 Histopathological features of odontoma. Irregular dentin tubules of complex odontoma

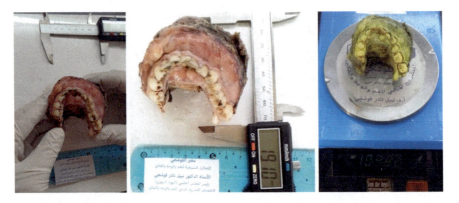

Fig. 2.36 Case of recurrent osteoma

2.4.2.2 Osteoma

Osteomas are benign neoplasms originating from bone and typically manifest as a well-defined radiopaque mass with smooth-surfaced radiopacities. They can occur in various regions of the jaws and are often asymptomatic. Its dense structure sets it apart, and its management is largely based on clinical symptoms and location. Surgical removal may be indicated if the osteoma is causing symptoms or significant esthetic concerns [4] (Fig. 2.36).

2.4.2.3 Cementoblastoma

Cementoblastomas are benign tumors that arise from the roots of teeth and are characterized by a radiopaque mass attached to the tooth root. They are typically associated with pain and tenderness. The lesion is well-defined and surrounded by a radiolucent halo. Surgical extraction of the affected tooth is usually required. This lesion is frequently associated with localized pain and necessitates careful assessment for optimal treatment planning [4].

2.4.2.4 Condensing Osteitis (Focal Sclerosing Osteomyelitis)

Condensing osteitis is a reactive bony change that occurs in response to chronic inflammation or infection. It presents as a localized area of increased bone density, often seen at the apex of a nonvital tooth. It is typically asymptomatic and does not require treatment unless associated with discomfort or other complications [9].

(Tip 13): With the widespread use of bisphosphonate in cancer patients, dentists are more frequently facing cases of osteomyelitis in modern dentistry compared to the practicing years ago.

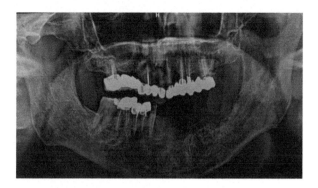

Fig. 2.37 Osteomyelitis on a patient under bisphosphonate treatment

2.4.2.5 Sclerosing Osteitis (Chronic Osteomyelitis)

Sclerosing osteitis is a chronic inflammatory condition that leads to increased bone density. It often presents as a radiopaque lesion surrounding the apex of a nonvital tooth and may be associated with a history of infection or trauma. Treatment focuses on addressing the underlying cause and may involve endodontic therapy or extraction [9] (Fig. 2.37).

2.4.2.6 Paget's Disease

Paget's disease is a chronic bone disorder that can affect the jaws. It results in abnormal bone remodeling and presents as a mixed radiolucent-radiopaque lesion with irregular borders. Additional signs, such as bone expansion and cotton-wool appearance, may be present. Treatment may involve medication and management of symptoms [9].

It's important to note that this is not an exhaustive list, and there can be other less common causes of radiopaque lesions in the jaws. A comprehensive evaluation, including clinical and radiographic examination, along with appropriate diagnostic tests and often a biopsy, is necessary for an accurate diagnosis and appropriate management of radiopaque jaw lesions.

2.4.3 Algorithm for Differential Diagnosis

This text aims to provide an algorithm of logical thinking to facilitate a comprehensive differential diagnosis for radiopaque lesions in the jaws.

Step 1: Repeat Steps 1 and 2
Step 2: Categorize Lesion Characteristics
Group lesions based on their radiographic characteristics [1]:

1. Pure radiopaque lesions with the same density as surrounding structures
2. Pure radiopaque lesions with different densities compared to surrounding structures
3. Mixed radiopaque lesions

Step 3: Consider Clinical Findings

1. Perform a thorough intraoral and extraoral examination to detect any swelling, erythema, ulceration, or bony expansion related to the lesion.
2. Evaluate the presence of associated symptoms such as pain, sensitivity, or mobility of adjacent teeth.

Step 4: Common Entities for Each Category

List the most common lesions associated with each category based on radiographic and clinical findings.

1. Pure radiopaque lesions with the same density as surrounding structures: odontoma, cementoblastoma, and osteoma (Fig. 2.38) [5]

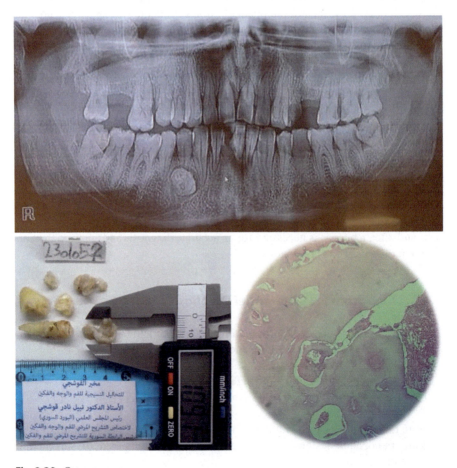

Fig. 2.38 Osteoma case

2. Pure radiopaque lesions with different densities compared to surrounding structures: ossifying fibroma, osseous dysplasia, and fibrous dysplasia [5]
3. Mixed radiopaque lesions: ossifying fibroma, cementoblastoma, calcifying odontogenic cyst (Gorlin cyst), and Pindborg tumor [5]

Step 5: Repeat Steps from 8 to 11

(Tip 14): In conclusion, radiopaque lesions encountered in the jaws encompass a wide spectrum of conditions with varying clinical implications. Precise diagnosis is pivotal in ensuring optimal patient care and determining the most suitable treatment approach. By understanding the attributes of prevalent lesions such as osteoma, cementoblastoma, and complex odontoma, and following a structured diagnostic algorithm, oral health professionals are empowered to provide accurate diagnoses and effective management plans for individuals presenting with radiopaque jaw lesions.

2.5 Categorization and Comprehensive Classification of Intraosseous Radiopaque Lesions in the Jaws

Introduction: Intraosseous radiopaque lesions within the jaws encompass a heterogeneous group of pathological entities that manifest as areas of increased radiodensity on radiographic imaging. These lesions arise due to a multitude of etiological factors, resulting in a wide spectrum of clinical presentations. Accurate categorization and classification of these lesions are pivotal for facilitating precise diagnosis, formulation of effective treatment strategies, and management of patient care.

2.5.1 Benign Neoplastic Lesions

2.5.1.1 Odontogenic Lesions
1. *Odontoma*: A developmental odontogenic anomaly resulting from aberrant dental tissue growth. Radiographically, it appears as a radiopaque mass with discernible internal structures resembling tooth-like components [4].

2.5.1.2 Nonodontogenic Lesions
1. *Osteoma*: A benign neoplasm primarily composed of compact or cancellous bone tissue. Radiographically, osteomas are identified as sharply circumscribed radiopacities, often occurring in the craniofacial region [4].
2. *Cemento-Osseous Dysplasia*: A fibro-osseous lesion categorized into different subtypes (periapical, focal, and florid) based on its location and extent. Radiographically, it demonstrates radiopaque regions, frequently encircled by a radiolucent halo [4].

2.5.2 Fibro-Osseous Lesions

2.5.2.1 Fibrous Dysplasia
A developmental disorder characterized by the replacement of normal bone with fibrous tissue and immature woven bone. Radiographs exhibit a ground-glass appearance due to the presence of irregularly distributed radiopacities (Fig. 2.39) [4].

2.5.2.2 Paget's Disease of Bone
A chronic metabolic disorder impacting bone remodeling processes. Radiographically, affected areas show a mosaic pattern of increased radiodensity, resembling a "cotton-wool" appearance [9].

2.5.3 Metabolic and Systemic Conditions

2.5.3.1 Hyperparathyroidism
Elevated parathyroid hormone levels lead to increased bone resorption and deposition, culminating in a speckled radiopacity pattern resembling "salt-and-pepper" on radiographs [9].

2.5.3.2 Renal Osteodystrophy
Skeletal changes associated with chronic kidney disease are evident radiographically through a medley of radiolucent and radiopaque areas, reflecting the complex interplay of mineral metabolism [9].

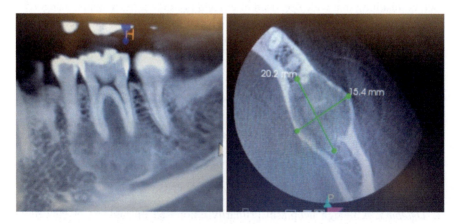

Fig. 2.39 Case of fibrous dysplasia, discovered accidentally on a radiograph

2.5.4 Malignant Lesions

2.5.4.1 Osteosarcoma
A malignant bone-forming tumor characterized by aggressive osteoid production and bone destruction. Radiographs typically display ill-defined radiopaque masses intertwined with radiolucent regions [4].

2.5.4.2 Chondrosarcoma
A malignancy arising from cartilaginous tissue, often presenting as variable radiodensity lesions, encompassing both radiopaque and radiolucent zones [4].

2.5.5 Developmental and Anatomical Variants

2.5.5.1 Torus Palatinus/Mandibularis
Benign bony protuberances occurring on the midline of the palate or lingual aspect of the mandible. Radiographically, they manifest as smooth radiopaque masses [9].

2.5.5.2 Accessory and Supernumerary Teeth
Additional teeth emerging in various jaw regions, contributing to localized radiopaque appearances [9] (Fig. 2.40 shows a rare case of bilateral ossifying fibroma).

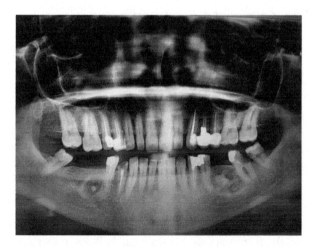

Fig. 2.40 Bilateral ossifying fibroma

(Tip 15): **In summary,** the meticulous categorization and classification of intraosseous radiopaque lesions in the jaws form the cornerstone of precise clinical diagnosis and the establishment of tailored treatment plans. A profound comprehension of the diverse range of lesions, their distinct radiographic characteristics, and the underlying pathogenic mechanisms is imperative for healthcare practitioners. Such understanding empowers clinicians to deliver optimal patient care, orchestrating interventions and therapies that align with the specific lesion category, ultimately enhancing patient outcomes and quality of life.

2.5.6 Vital Teeth

If a radiopaque lesion is attached to a vital tooth, the differential diagnosis may include the following conditions:

2.5.6.1 Dental Calculus (Calcified Plaque)

Dental calculus appears as mineralized deposits on the tooth surface, typically near the gingival margin or interproximal spaces. It presents as irregular radiopaque masses. Calculus can often be identified by its location and characteristic appearance [9].

2.5.6.2 Dental Cementum Hyperplasia

Cementum hyperplasia refers to excessive cementum formation on the roots of teeth. It appears as a localized radiopaque mass along the root surface. This condition is typically asymptomatic and does not require treatment unless it causes esthetic or functional concerns [9].

2.5.6.3 Condensing Osteitis

Condensing osteitis can also present as a radiopaque lesion associated with a vital tooth. It is a reactive bony change in response to chronic inflammation. The lesion appears as an area of increased bone density around the apex of a vital tooth. No specific treatment is required unless associated with symptoms or complications [9].

2.5.6.4 Hypercementosis

Hypercementosis refers to excessive cementum formation on the root surface of a tooth. It appears as a localized, bulbous radiopaque enlargement of the root. Hypercementosis is often associated with underlying factors such as trauma or chronic occlusal stress but typically does not require treatment unless causing functional issues or esthetic concerns [9].

2.5.6.5 Amalgam Restoration or Other Dental Materials

Radiopaque areas may be observed if the tooth has undergone restorative procedures using materials such as dental amalgam or other radiopaque restorative materials. The appearance and location of the radiopacity should correspond to the dental restoration [1, 5].

> (Tip 16): It is important to consider the clinical history, symptoms, and radiographic findings to arrive at an accurate diagnosis. In cases where the nature of the radiopaque lesion is uncertain or causing concerns, further evaluation by an oral and maxillofacial radiologist or consultation with an oral and maxillofacial surgeon may be beneficial for a definitive diagnosis and appropriate management.

2.5.7 Nonvital Teeth

If the radiopaque lesion is attached to a nonvital tooth, the differential diagnosis may include the following conditions:

2.5.7.1 Condensing Osteitis

Condensing osteitis, also known as chronic osteomyelitis, can occur in association with nonvital teeth. It presents as a localized area of increased bone density around the apex of the affected tooth. It is typically a reactive process in response to chronic inflammation or infection. Treatment may involve endodontic therapy, extraction, or management of the underlying cause [9].

2.5.7.2 Root Canal Filling Material

Radiopaque materials used for root canal filling, such as gutta-percha or other filling materials, can appear as radiopaque masses within the root canal space. The location and appearance of the radiopacity should correspond to the previously performed root canal treatment [1].

2.5.7.3 Dystrophic Calcifications

Dystrophic calcifications can occur in the pulp chamber or root canal space of nonvital teeth. These calcifications can result from pulp necrosis or chronic inflammation. Treatment may involve endodontic therapy or extraction if symptomatic or associated with complications [5, 21].

2.5.7.4 Cementoblastoma

Although rare, cementoblastomas can occur in association with nonvital teeth. They present as well-defined, radiopaque masses attached to the root surface. These tumors are typically associated with pain and require surgical extraction of the affected tooth [4].

(Tip 17): Accurate diagnosis often requires clinical evaluation, radiographic examination, and possibly histopathological examination through biopsy or surgical excision. Consultation with an endodontist, oral and maxillofacial surgeon, or a pathologist is recommended for an accurate diagnosis and appropriate management of radiopaque lesions associated with nonvital teeth.

2.5.8 Edentulous Area

If a radiopaque lesion is located in an edentulous area (an area without teeth), the differential diagnosis may include the following conditions:

2.5.8.1 Torus Mandibularis or Torus Palatinus
These are benign bony growths that can occur in the mandible (torus mandibularis) or the palate (torus palatinus). They present as smooth, bony protuberances and are typically asymptomatic. No treatment is necessary unless they cause functional or esthetic concerns [9].

2.5.8.2 Exostosis
Exostosis is the formation of bony outgrowths on the alveolar ridge or the mandible. It can occur as a response to mechanical stress or chronic irritation, such as wearing ill-fitting dentures. Exostoses are usually asymptomatic and may not require treatment unless they interfere with prosthodontic rehabilitation or cause discomfort [9].

2.5.8.3 Retained Root or Tooth Fragment
In some cases, a retained root or tooth fragment from a previously extracted tooth may be seen as a radiopaque mass in an edentulous area. This can occur if the tooth is not fully removed during the extraction procedure. Evaluation and possible removal of the retained fragment may be necessary if it causes discomfort or affects prosthodontic rehabilitation [22].

2.5.8.4 Calcified Lymph Nodes
Calcification or mineralization of lymph nodes can sometimes be seen on radiographs. These calcifications may appear as radiopaque masses in the edentulous area. Evaluation by a healthcare professional may be necessary to determine the significance of the calcified lymph nodes and rule out any underlying pathology [23].

2.5.8.5 Dystrophic Calcifications
Dystrophic calcifications can occur in soft tissues, such as blood vessels or salivary glands. These calcifications can appear as radiopaque masses on radiographs. Evaluation by a healthcare professional, including biopsy if necessary, may be required to determine the nature and significance of the calcifications [23].

2.5.8.6 Foreign Body

In rare cases, a radiopaque mass in an edentulous area may be due to the presence of a foreign body, such as a metallic or radiopaque object that was accidentally embedded during a previous procedure or trauma. Identification and removal of the foreign body may be necessary if it causes symptoms or concerns [24].

(Tip 18): Accurate diagnosis of a radiopaque lesion in an edentulous area often requires a thorough clinical evaluation, radiographic examination, and, if necessary, consultation with an oral and maxillofacial radiologist or oral and maxillofacial surgeon. Further diagnostic tests or procedures, such as biopsy or imaging, may be recommended to establish a definitive diagnosis and determine the appropriate management approach.

2.6 Differential Diagnosis of a Mixed Radiolucent/ Radiopaque Lesion in the Jaws (Algorithm of Logic Thinking)

Mixed radiolucent/radiopaque lesions in the jaws present a diagnostic challenge due to their diverse etiologies and overlapping radiographic appearances. This coming paragraph proposes an algorithm of logical thinking to aid in the differential diagnosis of such lesions. The algorithm systematically guides clinicians through a series of steps to arrive at the most probable diagnosis based on radiographic findings, clinical features, and patient history. Accurate identification of these lesions is crucial for appropriate management and improved patient outcomes.

2.6.1 Introduction

Mixed radiolucent/radiopaque lesions in the jaws are less commonly encountered in dental and maxillofacial practice compared to radiolucent lesions. These lesions appear as areas of varying radiopacity on radiographs, exhibiting both radiolucent (dark) and radiopaque (light) components. Due to their heterogeneous nature, differential diagnosis becomes complex, necessitating a systematic approach for accurate identification. This text aims to provide a logical algorithm to facilitate a comprehensive differential diagnosis for these challenging lesions.

2.6.2 Top Frequent Mixed Lesions

With bearing in mind all differential diagnoses presented as possibilities in radiopaque lesions, we can add:

2.6.2.1 Adenomatoid Odontogenic Tumor (AOT)

AOT is a benign, slow-growing tumor associated with impacted teeth. It often presents as a radiolucent lesion with small radiopaque flecks, resembling a "soap bubble" appearance [4].

2.6.2.2 Calcifying Epithelial Odontogenic Tumor (CEOT)

CEOT is a rare odontogenic tumor that may exhibit mixed radiolucent-radiopaque features. Radiographically, it can show calcifications within a radiolucent lesion [4].

2.6.3 Algorithm for Differential Diagnosis

The following algorithm outlines a step-by-step logical approach to differentiate and diagnose mixed radiolucent/radiopaque lesions in the jaws:

Step 1: Repeat Steps 1 and 2 from the general algorithm
Step 2: Review the panoramic or intraoral radiographs
to identify the presence of mixed radiolucent/radiopaque lesions.

1. Note the precise location and borders of the lesion.
2. Assess the density and pattern of radiolucency and radiopacity within the lesion.

Step 3: Categorize Lesion Characteristics
Group lesions into three main categories based on predominant features [1]:

1. Radiolucent-dominant lesions with minor radiopaque elements.
2. Radiopaque-dominant lesions with minor radiolucent elements.
3. Equally mixed radiolucent/radiopaque lesions.

Step 4: Consider Clinical Findings

1. Perform a thorough intraoral and extraoral examination to detect any swelling, erythema, ulceration, or bony expansion.
2. Evaluate the presence of associated symptoms such as pain, paresthesia, or mobility of adjacent teeth.

Step 5: Common Entities for Each Category
List the most common lesions associated with each category based on radiographic and clinical findings.

1. Radiolucent-dominant lesions: central giant cell granuloma [5].
2. Radiopaque-dominant lesions: ossifying fibroma, cementoblastoma, and osteoma [5].
3. Equally mixed lesions: complex odontoma, compound odontoma, and cemento-ossifying fibroma [5].

Step 6: Rare Entities and Differential Diagnosis

1. Enumerate less common lesions and entities that may present with mixed radiolucent/radiopaque appearances.
2. Consider systemic conditions that may manifest as jaw lesions, such as Paget's disease, fibrous dysplasia, or hyperparathyroidism [5].

Step 7: Repeat Steps 8 to 11

> (Tip 19): The algorithm of logical thinking presented in this text serves as a valuable tool for clinicians in diagnosing mixed radiolucent/radiopaque lesions in the jaws. By carefully considering patient history, radiographic findings, clinical features, and auxiliary investigations, dental and maxillofacial professionals can accurately differentiate these lesions and implement appropriate treatment plans for improved patient care.

2.6.4 Vital Teeth

When dealing with mixed radiolucent/radiopaque lesions attached to vital teeth, the diagnostic approach should be even more meticulous. By considering the relationship between the lesion and the vital tooth, clinicians can make well-informed decisions about the diagnosis and management, aiming to preserve the tooth's health and function while addressing the underlying pathology.

Most common lesions encountered are:

2.6.4.1 Pindborg Tumor

Pindborg tumor, also known as Calcifying Epithelial Odontogenic Tumor (CEOT), is a rare odontogenic tumor originating from the epithelial tissue associated with teeth. It typically presents as a slow-growing lesion within the jawbones, often the mandible. Radiographically, it may exhibit a mixed radiolucent-radiopaque appearance due to calcifications within a predominantly radiolucent lesion. Pindborg tumors are generally benign but can be locally aggressive. Surgical removal is the standard treatment, and long-term follow-up is essential to monitor for potential recurrence (Fig. 2.41) [4].

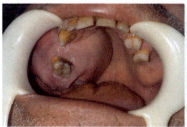 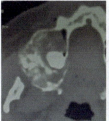 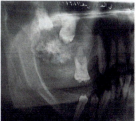

Fig. 2.41 Delay of diagnosis of Pindborg tumor

2.6.5 Nonvital Teeth

Based on the differential diagnosis and the impact on the nonvital tooth, determine the most appropriate treatment plan. This may involve surgical excision, endodontic treatment, or extraction of the nonvital tooth, depending on the specific diagnosis and clinical situation.

When dealing with mixed radiolucent/radiopaque lesions attached to nonvital teeth, the diagnostic approach remains meticulous. Considering the impact on the nonvital tooth, clinicians can make well-informed decisions about the diagnosis and management, aiming to address the underlying pathology while ensuring the best possible outcome for the patient's oral health and overall well-being.

2.6.6 Edentulous Area

Based on the differential diagnosis and the location in the edentulous area, determine the most appropriate treatment plan. This may involve surgical excision or other interventions, depending on the specific diagnosis and clinical situation.

> (Tip 20): When dealing with mixed radiolucent/radiopaque lesions in edentulous areas, the diagnostic approach should consider the absence of teeth and the potential implications for adjacent structures. By thoroughly evaluating the radiographic and clinical features and considering the differential diagnosis, clinicians can make informed decisions about the management of these lesions, aiming to address the underlying pathology and maintain the overall health and function of the edentulous region.

2.7 Summary of Part Two

Commonly, in dentistry, it is believed that the healing lesion seen on radiographs as a unilocular radiolucent lesion can be one of three things: periapical granuloma, radicular cyst, or dentigerous cyst, depending on its size and its relationship to the tooth.

In the upcoming algorithm, I will attempt to correct this common and deadly mistake! Please continue and refer to the paragraph numbers.

Is the lesion associated with a tooth?
1. (Yes, the lesion is associated with a tooth)
    (a) Is the tooth erupted? (Yes, it is erupted):
        - Is it vital?
            - (Yes, it is vital) please refer to paragraph: Sect. 2.2.4
            - (No, it is not vital) please refer to paragraph: Sect. 2.2.5
    (b) (No, it is not erupted): please refer to paragraph: Sect. 2.2.7

2.7 Summary of Part Two

2. (No): The lesion is not associated with the tooth.
    Is the tooth extracted, missing, or is the lesion away from the tooth area?
    (a) (Tooth is extracted) here, we omit the radicular cyst.
    (b) (Tooth is missing) here, we omit the dentigerous cyst and the differential diagnosis here, in addition to all cysts, tumors, and cancers mentioned in paragraph Sect. 2.2.7, is a primordial cyst, which is histologically one of the types of odontogenic keratocysts. Please refer to paragraph Sect. 4.3.3.
    (c) (Lesion is away from the tooth area) in addition to lesions described in paragraph: Sect. 2.2.6
       - Nasopalatine cyst
       - Median palatal cyst
       - Nasolabial cyst (paragraph: Sect. 3.2)
       - Hematopoietic benign tumors (to be discussed in rare lesions paragraph: Sect. 4.4)
         Practical Application of Logical Thinking Algorithm.

2.7.1 Lesion Seen on Radiographs as a Unilocular Radiolucent Lesion on an Erupted and Vital Tooth

2.7.1.1 Most Common and Benign Lesions
- Odontogenic keratocyst
- Ameloblastoma in its various forms
- Odontogenic glandular cyst
- Paradontal cyst
- Odontogenic myxoma

2.7.1.2 Less Common Lesions
- Cementoblastoma (in its early stages)
- Pindborg tumor
- Plasmacytoma (Fig. 2.42)
- Intraosseous cancers

The lesion is seen on radiographs as a unilocular radiolucent lesion on an erupted and nonvital tooth.

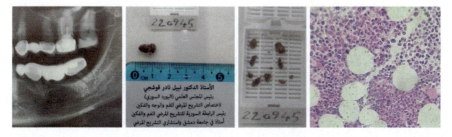

Fig. 2.42 A lesion that was frequently described as a residual cyst turned out to be a plasmacytoma!

In addition to the lesions mentioned in paragraph Sect. 2.7.1.1, the differential diagnosis of a unilocular radiolucent lesion associated with an erupted nonvital tooth also includes:

- Granuloma (around the apex or lateral area).
- Radicular cyst (in any of its three patterns).

(Tip 21): Important Note: In multi-rooted teeth, a granuloma may develop and transform into a radicular cyst at the expense of one of the root canals, while the tooth continues to show vital signs due to the presence of live canals in the other roots. This is not a common condition but is possible.

2.7.2 Lesion Seen on Radiographs as a Unilocular Radiolucent Lesion on a Nonerupted Tooth

(Tip 22): First, it must be remembered that a nonerupted tooth is not necessarily an impacted tooth; it may be an embedded tooth, where part of it has erupted into the oral cavity while the other part failed to erupt and remains embedded. This is most common in the lower third molars.

The differential diagnosis of a unilocular radiolucent lesion associated with a nonerupted tooth includes all cysts, tumors, and cancers mentioned in Benefits Sect. 2.7.1.1, plus:

- Dentigerous cyst.

(Tip 23): Dentigerous cyst accounts for no more than 60% of these lesions. It is a prerequisite for differential diagnosis that it be attached to the anatomical neck of the tooth or, if it is large and surrounds the entire tooth. It should be excluded from differential diagnosis if the lesion is located only at the unerupted tooth's roots.

(Tip 24): When saying "missing tooth," we do not mean a tooth that the patient extracted and forgot about. We do mean a tooth that has never developed and the most common example of this is a missing third molar, which may present as a lesion seen on radiographs as a unilocular radiolucent lesion.

References

1. Iannucci J, Howerton LJ. Dental radiography—e-book: principles and techniques. Elsevier Health Sciences; 2016.
2. Regezi JA, Sciubba J, Jordan RC. Oral pathology: clinical pathologic correlations. Elsevier Health Sciences; 2016.
3. Hardiman R, Kujan O, Kochaji N. Normal variation in the anatomy, biology, and histology of the maxillofacial region. Contemporary oral medicine: a comprehensive approach to clinical practice. Springer International Publishing AG; 2019. p. 1–66.
4. El-Naggar AK, Chan JKC, Grandis JR, Takata T, Slootweg PJ. WHO classification of head and neck tumours. International Agency for Research on Cancer; 2017.
5. Regezi JA, Sciubba J, Jordan RCK. Oral pathology—e-book: oral pathology—e-book. Elsevier Health Sciences; 2011.
6. Shear M, Speight PM. Cysts of the oral and maxillofacial regions. John Wiley & Sons; 2008.
7. Stajčić Z, Paljm A. Keratinization of radicular cyst epithelial lining or occurrence of odontogenic keratocyst in the periapical region? Int J Oral Maxillofac Surg. 1987;16(5):593–5.
8. Kashyap B, Reddy PS, Desai RS. Plexiform ameloblastoma mimicking a periapical lesion: a diagnostic dilemma. J Conserv Dent. 2012;15(1):84.
9. Neville BW, Damm DD, Allen CM, Chi AC. Oral and maxillofacial pathology. Elsevier Health Sciences; 2023.
10. Dahlkemper P, Wolcott JF, Pringle GA, Hicks ML. Periapical central giant cell granuloma: a potential endodontic misdiagnosis. Oral Surg Oral Med Oral Pathol Oral Radiol Endod. 2000;90(6):739–45.
11. Farah C, Balasubramaniam R, McCullough MJ. Contemporary oral medicine. Springer; 2019.
12. Erasmus J, Thompson I, Van Rensburg L, Van der Westhuijzen A. Central calcifying odontogenic cyst. A review of the literature and the role of advanced imaging techniques. Dentomaxillofac Radiol. 1998;27(1):30–5.
13. Kochaji N, Darwich K, Ahmad M, Mahfuri A. Bilateral ossifying fibroma affecting the jaws: literature review, rare case report. Int J Surg Case Rep. 2023;106:108283.
14. Kochaji N, Goossens A, Bottenberg P. Central Mucoepidermoid carcinoma: case report, literature review for missing and available information and guideline proposal for coming case reports. Oral Oncol Extra. 2004;40(8–9):95–105.
15. Veena K, Rao R, Jagadishchandra H, Rao PK. Odontogenic keratocyst looks can be deceptive, causing endodontic misdiagnosis. Case Rep Pathol. 2011;2011:159501.
16. Figueiredo NR, Meena M, Dinkar AD, Malik S, Khorate M. Unicystic ameloblastoma presenting as a multilocular radiolucency in the anterior mandible: a case report. J Dent Res Dent Clin Dent Prospects. 2015;9(3):199.
17. Choi Y-J, Oh S-H, Kang J-H, Choi H-Y, Kim G-T, Yu J-J, et al. Primary intraosseous squamous cell carcinoma mimicking periapical disease: a case report. Imaging Sci Dent. 2012;42(4):265–70.
18. Shah M, Kale H, Ranginwala A, Patel G. Glandular odontogenic cyst: a rare entity. J Oral Maxillofac Pathol. 2014;18(1):89.
19. Kochaji N, Alhessani S, Ibrahim S, Al-Awad A. Posterior mandibular glandular cyst: a rare case report. Int J Surg Case Rep. 2023;106:108169.
20. Ahuja P, Rathore AS, Chhina S, Manchanda A. Aggressive central giant cell granuloma mimicking giant cell tumor. IJCRI. 2011;2(2):5–10.
21. Odell EW. Cawson's essentials of oral pathology and oral medicine e-book: Cawson's essentials of oral pathology and oral medicine e-book. Elsevier Health Sciences; 2017.
22. Karjodkar FR. Essentials of oral & maxillofacial radiology. Jaypee Brothers Medical Publishers Pvt. Limited; 2019.
23. Omami G. Soft tissue calcification in oral and maxillofacial imaging: a pictorial review. Int J Dent Oral Sci. 2016;3(4):219–24.
24. Kose TE, Demirtas N, Karabas HC, Ozcan I. Evaluation of dental panoramic radiographic findings in edentulous jaws: a retrospective study of 743 patients. J Adv Prosthodont. 2015;7(5):380–5.

All Intraosseous Lesion of the Jaws

3

Frankly when I wanted to write this part of the book, I had to choose whether to order the lists of all the diseases and lesions previously mentioned through the first and second part alphabetically or in their frequency.

Later I decided to list them into six categories, and to order them from more to less frequent. The deferential diagnosis is discussed in Chap. 2, but here we are going to list all intraosseous lesion starting from more to less frequent lesions as possible:

The description will focus on clinical relevant information and the histological description will be minimum.

We can start a routine introduction by listing all classification of intraosseous lesions in the jaws.

They are categorized into six groups:

1. Odontogenic cysts.
2. Non-odontogenic cysts.
3. Odontogenic tumors.
4. Non-odontogenic tumors.
5. Intraosseous primary malignancies.
6. Metastatic malignancies.

3.1 Odontogenic Cysts

3.1.1 Introduction

Odontogenic cysts represent a diverse group of lesions that develop within the oral and maxillofacial region. These cysts are of paramount importance in the fields of dentistry and oral medicine due to their potential to cause significant morbidity if left untreated. Understanding the various types, methods of diagnosis, and appropriate management strategies is essential for dental and medical practitioners.

© The Author(s), under exclusive license to Springer Nature Switzerland AG 2024
N. Kochaji, *Clinical Oral Pathology*,
https://doi.org/10.1007/978-3-031-53755-4_3

3.1.2 Definition of Odontogenic Cysts

Odontogenic cysts are pathological fluid-filled cavities lined by odontogenic epithelium [1].

Odontogenic cysts are a group of cystic lesions that arise from the epithelial remnants associated with tooth development. These cysts are primarily found in the jaws and are often classified based on their origin, such as developmental or inflammatory etiology. The most common types of odontogenic cysts include *radicular cysts*, *dentigerous cysts*, and *odontogenic keratocysts* [2, 3].

Odontogenic cysts typically present as painless, slow-growing swellings in the jaw region. They may be discovered incidentally on routine dental radiographs or during evaluation for other dental or maxillofacial concerns [3, 4].

> (Tip 1): Unless odontogenic cysts are infected or suffered from malignant transformation, they remain silent.

Radiographically, these cysts appear as well-defined radiolucent lesions, often in the tooth-bearing area. Histologically, odontogenic cysts exhibit a lining of stratified squamous epithelium (differs between types, and is essential for final diagnosis), and the cystic space may contain inflammatory cells or (sometimes) keratinous material [5].

Radicular cysts are the most common type of odontogenic cyst and arise as a result of pulpal inflammation or necrosis, associated with a non-vital tooth.

Dentigerous cysts, also known as follicular cysts, develop around the crown of an unerupted or impacted tooth and are typically associated with the crown of a partially erupted third molar.

Odontogenic keratocysts, on the other hand, are known for their aggressive behavior and high recurrence rate. They often present as large, multilocular lesions and have a propensity for infiltrating the surrounding tissues [6].

3.1.3 Importance in Dentistry and Oral Medicine

Odontogenic cysts represent the top frequent intraosseous lesions that general dentist might face in his daily practice [3].

Due to the fifty two tooth germs that evolve in both jaws, a lot of silent/inactive odontogenic epithelial remnant cells are scattered all over the osseous structure of the jaws. These include the following:

1. **Remnant of Serres:**

    Epithelial cells, firstly described by Serres, represent the reduced epithelium of the dental lamina [7].

    They are claimed as the responsible source of odontogenic keratocysts and varies types of ameloblastomas [8].

3.1 Odontogenic Cysts

2. **Rests of Malassez:**

   Epithelial cells, firstly described by Malassez, represent the reduced epithelium of Hertwig Sheath [9].

   They are proven as the responsible source of radicular cyst with all its three subtypes, and of periimplant cyst [8, 10].

3. **Reduced Enamel Epithelium:**

   Two layers of epithelial cells represent the reduced enamel epithelium that covers the teeth crown till eruption is completed [11].

   They are accused as the responsible source of dentigerous cysts [8].

3.1.4 Classification of Odontogenic Cysts

3.1.4.1 Developmental Cysts

1. **Dentigerous Cyst:**

   This is one of the most common odontogenic cysts and typically forms as a result of the accumulation of fluid between the crown of an unerupted tooth and the reduced enamel epithelium that covers the crown. It is often associated with impacted third molars and can cause expansion of the jaw [12].

2. **Odontogenic Keratocyst (OKC):**

   OKCs are known for their locally aggressive behavior, high recurrence rates, and a predilection for occurring in the posterior mandible. Understanding their pathogenesis and management is crucial due to their challenging nature. Their special concern comes from their tendency to recurrence; this is accused by two unique histological features: daughter cysts that might exist in the connective tissue, and epithelial separation [12].

3. **Calcifying Odontogenic Cyst (Gorlin Cyst):**

   This cyst is characterized by the presence of calcifications and various histological features, often mimicking other lesions. It is associated with the nevoid basal cell carcinoma syndrome [12].

4. **Lateral Periodontal Cyst:**

   Typically found between the roots of vital teeth, lateral periodontal cysts are relatively small but can lead to bone resorption and should not be overlooked [12].

> (Tip 2): Never try to diagnose the radiolucency, it can only give differential diagnosis.

3.1.4.2 Inflammatory Cysts

1. **Radicular Cyst:**

   These cysts develop as a result of chronic inflammation in the periapical region of a non-vital tooth. Early diagnosis and endodontic treatment are essential to prevent their formation [12].

2. **Residual Cyst:**
   Residual cyst is subtype of radicular cyst, occurs when the initiating tooth is extracted and a radicular cyst is not completely removed during treatment or when the cystic lining is left behind. Monitoring and additional surgical intervention may be necessary [12, 13].
3. **Periimplant Cyst:**
   An inflammatory odontogenic cyst was first fully described and reported in 2017. These cysts are typically formed due to inflammatory process in the bone surrounding a dental implant that activates the epithelial remnants. Periimplant cysts are often asymptomatic in their early stages, making them challenging to detect without regular dental check-ups and imaging. However, if left untreated, they can lead to complications such as implant failure, bone loss, and even damage to adjacent teeth [10].

3.1.4.3 Other Rare Developmental Odontogenic Cysts
1. **Glandular Odontogenic Cyst:**
   A rare entity characterized by its complex histological features and potential for aggressive behavior (Fig. 3.1) [12].
2. **Orthokeratinized Odontogenic Cyst:**
   This cyst is similar in appearance to the OKC but tends to have a less aggressive and less recurrence tendency clinical course [12].

3.1.5 Etiology and Pathogenesis

The development of odontogenic cysts is multifactorial and involves interactions between genetic, molecular, and environmental factors. Dental follicles play a crucial role in cyst formation. Certain genetic mutations and molecular markers have been associated with the development of odontogenic keratocysts, providing insights into their pathogenesis [14].

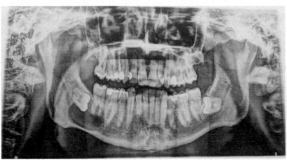
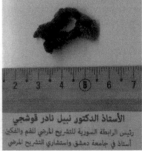

Fig. 3.1 Radiolucent lesion attached to impacted teeth. It looks like an innocent dentigerous cyst, on radiographs and even on macroscopic sectioning, but it is in fact glandular odontogenic cyst

3.1 Odontogenic Cysts

Inflammation is another key factor in the pathogenesis of odontogenic cysts, particularly in the case of radicular cysts. Chronic inflammation in the periapical region can stimulate the formation of these inflammatory cysts [8, 12, 15].

3.1.6 Cyst Formation and Growing

All odontogenic cysts whether developmental or inflammatory have the same method of formation, briefly [13, 15]:

1. A *trigger* activates silent inactive epithelial remnants and induces them to proliferate from single isolated cells to form an epithelial cellular mass.

> (Tip 3): The trigger that induces cyst formation is either inflammatory (inflammatory cysts), or unknown (developmental cysts).

2. Cells keep on **proliferating** and the centric epithelial cells undergo necrosis due to lack of blood supply.

> (Tip 4): Because epithelium by definition lacks direct blood supply, they are fed by absorption from nearby connective tissue and for that epithelial layers cannot exceed certain thickness.

3. A lumen is formed, lined by the epithelial cells, and filled with cellular debris from the necrotic cells, that's what we call it—*cyst*.

> (Tip 5): The epithelial lining proliferation continue to go on regardless from the trigger, that's why the so-called residual cyst keeps growing although its trigger (the infected tooth) has already been extracted.

4. Due to the gap created in the centric part of the cyst (the lumen), making hydrostatic pressure unstable, and due to continuous epithelial proliferation the cystic lesion grows.

3.1.7 Radiographic and Histological Features

Almost all odontogenic cysts are radiolucent unilocular lesions that make their diagnosis based on radiographical features next to impossible; still each type of odontogenic cyst has its unique histological view (Fig. 3.2).

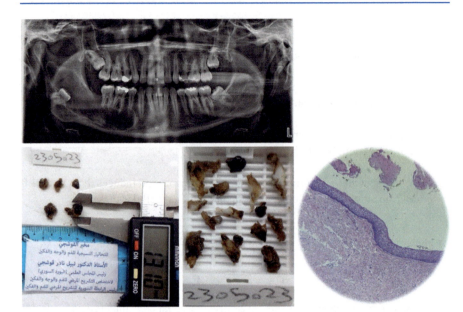

Fig. 3.2 A radiolucent lesion associated with impacted third molar. It could be any developmental odontogenic cyst or tumor. In this case final diagnosis was odontogenic keratocyst

> (Tip 6): The only certain and definitive diagnosis of odontogenic cysts should be based on histological features of the epithelial lining.

3.1.8 Clinical Presentation

Odontogenic cysts may present with a variety of symptoms and signs, depending on their size and location. Patients may report pain, swelling, or discomfort. On clinical examination, a palpable mass or expansion of the jaw may be evident. Radiographic radiolucencies discovered accidently might be the first sign of existence of an odontogenic cyst.

The clinical presentation of odontogenic cysts may include the following:

1. **Asymptomatic Lesions:** Many odontogenic cysts are discovered incidentally during routine dental or radiographic examinations. These asymptomatic cysts may not cause any noticeable symptoms, but they are typically detected through X-rays or imaging studies [12, 15].
2. **Swelling:** Odontogenic cysts can cause localized swelling in the jaw area. The size of the swelling may vary depending on the type of cyst and its growth rate. Swelling is often painless unless there is a secondary infection or inflammation [12, 15].

3. **Pain or Discomfort:** While odontogenic cysts are often painless, some patients may experience mild discomfort or a feeling of pressure in the affected area, especially if the cyst has grown significantly or if there is inflammation or infection [8].
4. **Tooth Mobility:** Cysts that develop in proximity to teeth can lead to tooth mobility or looseness. This occurs because the cyst erodes the surrounding bone and **affects** the tooth's stability [8, 13].
5. **Alterations in Occlusion:** In some cases, the presence of a cyst may cause changes in the way the teeth come together (occlusion). This can lead to bite irregularities or difficulty in chewing.
6. **Discharge or Fistula:** A long-standing cyst may create a path of least **resistance**, resulting in the formation of a fistula (an abnormal opening) in the overlying mucosa. This can lead to the discharge of fluid or pus into the mouth or through the skin [16].
7. **Gingival or Mucosal Changes:** Odontogenic cysts located in the maxilla can sometimes cause swelling or changes in the appearance of the gingiva or the **overlying** oral mucosa [13].
8. **Sinus Involvement:** Cysts in the upper jaw (maxillary sinus) may extend into the sinus **cavity**, potentially leading to symptoms such as sinus congestion, pain, or chronic sinusitis [17].
9. **Pathological Fractures:** In severe cases where the cyst has significantly **weakened** the jawbone, it can lead to pathological fractures, which are fractures that occur without significant trauma or injury [18].
10. **Secondary Infections:** Odontogenic cysts can become infected, resulting in localized pain, swelling, and tenderness. Infection can also lead to systemic symptoms like fever [13].

3.1.9 Radiographic Findings

Radiographic imaging, such as X-rays, panoramic radiographs, and cone-beam computed tomography (CBCT) scans, plays a crucial role in diagnosing odontogenic cysts. On imaging, these cysts typically appear as well-defined radiolucent areas within the bone.

It's important to note that the clinical presentation of odontogenic cysts can vary depending on the specific type of cyst (e.g., radicular cyst, dentigerous cyst, odontogenic keratocyst) and its location. Additionally, some cysts may remain asymptomatic for a long time before causing noticeable symptoms.

Early detection and appropriate management of odontogenic cysts are essential to prevent potential complications, such as tooth loss, bone destruction, and infection. Dentists and oral and maxillofacial surgeons play a key role in diagnosing and treating these cystic lesions.

3.1.10 Differential Diagnosis

As almost all odontogenic cysts are unilocular well-defined radiolucent lesions, they cannot be diagnosed from radiographs. But we have to keep in mind that:

(Tip 7): No radicular cyst without non-vital teeth.

(Tip 8): No dentigerous cyst without impacted teeth.

3.1.11 Final Diagnosis

Accurate diagnosis of odontogenic cysts relies on a combination of clinical, radiographic, and histopathological examinations. Panoramic radiography, cone-beam computed tomography (CBCT), magnetic resonance imaging (MRI), and ultrasonography are valuable tools for visualizing these lesions. Still histopathological examination of biopsy specimens remains the gold standard for definitive diagnosis.

In recent years, molecular markers, such as PTCH mutations in OKCs, have gained attention as diagnostic aids, offering a more precise understanding of the nature of these cysts [14].

3.1.12 Management and Treatment

The treatment of odontogenic cysts generally involves surgical intervention. The approach may vary depending on the size, location, and specific characteristics of the cyst. Surgical management typically includes enucleation or marsupialization of the cyst, with or without extraction of associated teeth. Histopathological examination of the cyst lining is essential to confirm the diagnosis and rule out other pathologies, such as odontogenic tumors.

While most odontogenic cysts are benign and treatable, they can cause significant morbidity if left untreated or if they recur. Regular follow-up and monitoring are important to detect any signs of recurrence or associated complications.

Additionally, appropriate dental management, such as endodontic treatment of non-vital teeth or extraction of impacted teeth associated with cysts, may be necessary to prevent recurrence or further complications.

The management of odontogenic cysts varies depending on the type, size, and location of the lesion. Several treatment options are available, including the following:

3.1.12.1 Conservative Treatment

1. **Enucleation and Curettage:** This is a common approach for smaller cysts. It involves the removal of the cystic lining and surrounding pathological tissue. Curettage helps ensure the complete elimination of cystic remnants [13].
2. **Marsupialization/Decompression:** In cases where cysts are large or removal may cause significant damage, marsupialization involves creating an opening in the cystic wall and allowing it to drain, promoting regression. Subsequent enucleation may be performed once the cyst has reduced in size [13].

3.1.12.2 Surgical Treatment

1. **En Bloc Resection:** Some aggressive or recurrent cysts may require en bloc resection, involving the complete removal of the cyst along with surrounding tissues. This approach is often employed for odontogenic keratocysts due to their higher recurrence rates [19, 20].

3.1.13 Management of Recurrent Cysts

Recurrence is a significant concern with certain types of odontogenic cysts, particularly odontogenic keratocysts. In such cases, careful monitoring and regular follow-up are essential. If a cyst recurs, more aggressive surgical techniques or adjunctive therapies, such as Carnoy's solution, may be considered to minimize the risk of further recurrence [15].

3.1.14 Adjunctive Therapies (e.g., Carnoy's Solution)

Carnoy's solution, a combination of ethanol, chloroform, and glacial acetic acid, has been used as an adjunctive therapy in the treatment of odontogenic keratocysts [21]. It is applied to the surgical site after the cyst removal; the rationale behind using Carnoy's solution in keratocyst surgery was to destroy the residual lining of the cyst and any potentially remaining cystic tissue at the surgical site. This was believed to decrease the chances of recurrence, which can be relatively high with keratocysts [21].

However, the use of Carnoy's solution in this context has diminished over time due to several factors, including concerns about its safety and its potential to cause damage to healthy tissues if not applied correctly. Additionally, there has been ongoing research to explore alternative treatment modalities for keratocysts, such as enucleation and adjunctive treatments like cryotherapy, bone grafting, and application of certain medications [21].

The decision to use Carnoy's solution in keratocyst surgery should be made based on a thorough evaluation of the patient's condition, taking into consideration the potential benefits and risks. It's essential for the surgical team to be well-trained in its proper application and to follow safety protocols to minimize risks associated with the solution's components, particularly chloroform. In many cases, surgeons may opt for alternative treatment strategies or techniques that do not involve the use of Carnoy's solution to achieve satisfactory results while prioritizing patient safety.

3.1.15 Follow-Up and Monitoring

Long-term follow-up is critical in the management of odontogenic cysts to monitor for any signs of recurrence or complications. Regular radiographic examinations are typically performed to ensure that the treated area remains healthy.

3.1.16 Complications and Their Management

Complications associated with odontogenic cysts can be categorized into four categories:

1. **Pathological Fractures:**
   It can occur if left untreated and reach huge sizes, or in patients that have potential bone fractures (Fig. 3.3) [13].
2. **Infection:**
   If treated poorly, especially the inflammatory types, and dentigerous cysts on partially erupted teeth [13].
3. **Neoplastic Transformation:**
   Developmental cysts have the ability to transform into benign tumors, mainly ameloblastomas (Figs. 3.3, 3.4) [8].
4. **Malignant Transformation:**
   The major complication is malignant transformation of odontogenic cyst. Central mucoepidermoid carcinoma cases have been reported (almost 200 cases) in the literature [22, 23]; they are thought to be a result of malignant transformation in the epithelial lining of a long persisting dentigerous cyst [8].
   Central squamous cell carcinoma cases (almost 250) have also been reported [24].

Prompt recognition, accurate diagnosis, and appropriate management of these complications are essential to minimize patient morbidity [1] (Fig. 3.5).

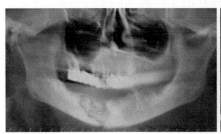
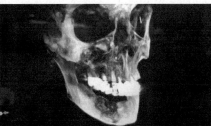

Fig. 3.3 Patient suffered from pathological fracture due to non-treated residual cyst

3.1 Odontogenic Cysts

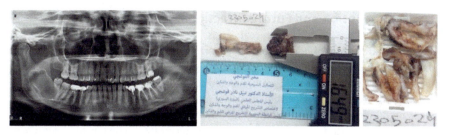

Fig. 3.4 Radiolucent lesion in the mandibular angle. Although it looks on radiographs and by macroscopic sectioning as a primordial cyst

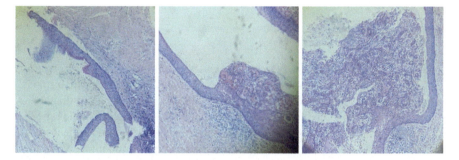

Fig. 3.5 Histopathological view of lesion in Fig. 3.4. The serial sectioning showed a benign neoplastic transformation in the epithelial cystic lining

3.1.17 Prognosis and Long-Term Outcomes

The prognosis for odontogenic cysts largely depends on early diagnosis and appropriate management. Besides the possibility of neoplastic transformation, with timely and effective treatment, the prognosis is generally favorable, and most patients can expect a full recovery. However, recurrent cysts, particularly in the case of odontogenic keratocysts, may require ongoing management and monitoring.

3.1.18 Odontogenic Cysts in Pediatric Dentistry

Special considerations are necessary when diagnosing and treating odontogenic cysts in pediatric patients. The impact on the developing dentition and jaws must be carefully evaluated, and treatment plans should be tailored to the child's growth and development.

Still common cystic lesions in adults such as radicular cyst are rare in children [15].

3.1.19 Prevention and Future Directions

Preventive strategies for odontogenic cysts primarily revolve around early detection and treatment of dental infections and pathology. Regular dental checkups, particularly for impacted or non-vital teeth, can aid in early diagnosis.

Ongoing research is essential to better understand the genetic and molecular basis of odontogenic cysts, leading to improved diagnostic tools and treatment options. Genetic studies and risk assessment may offer insights into identifying individuals at higher risk for certain cyst types.

Who knows! Genetic treatment might replace the surgical treatment approach. This might be a dream now, but a reality in the near future [1]!

3.1.20 Conclusion

(Tip 9): In summary, odontogenic cysts are a diverse group of cystic lesions that arise from remnants of the dental apparatus. They can present a diagnostic and therapeutic challenge, requiring careful evaluation, histopathological examination, and appropriate surgical management for optimal patient outcomes. A thorough understanding of the various types of odontogenic cysts and their clinical, radiographic, and histological features is essential for accurate diagnosis and effective treatment planning.

(Tip 10): Never judge cortical bone from 3D CBCT! (Fig. 3.6).

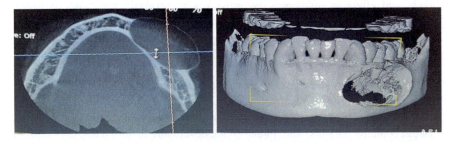

Fig. 3.6 Two images for the same odontogenic cyst. Note that in CT scan image the cortical bone was expanded and preserved, and not penetrated, while 3D CBCT showed an illusion of cortical bone penetration

3.2 Non-odontogenic Cysts

3.2.1 Introduction

Non-odontogenic cysts within the jaws are cystic lesions that develop in the bone and soft tissues of the oral cavity, excluding those associated with the teeth. These cysts can result from a variety of factors, such as developmental anomalies, inflammation, or trauma to the jaw area [25]. Diagnosis and management of these jaw-related non-odontogenic cysts are essential to prevent potential complications, which may include pain, bone loss, or interference with dental and facial structures.

3.2.2 Definition of Non-odontogenic Cysts

The true (epithelial lined) cysts originate from an epithelium not related to tooth development.

Historically they were named "Fissural" as they are located at the fusion line of the fissures responsible of maxillofacial complex formation [8].

Fissural cysts used to be classified into five types [26]:

1. Naso-labial.
2. Naso-platine.
3. Globular.
4. Median palatine (incisive canal cyst).
5. Median mandibular.

But in the last three decades and among immunohistochemistry wide application, that helped in exact determination of the origin of each cell, only naso-labial cyst and incisive canal cyst among all the five categories are accepted in recent claccification to be non-odontogenic cysts.

Other less frequent cysts of non-odontogenic origin include [25]:

1. Epidermal cyst.
2. Stafne cyst.
3. Solitary bone cyst.
4. Aneurysmal bone cyst.

(Tip 11): All non-odontogenic cysts are developmental; none of them is inflammatory.

3.2.3 Importance in Dentistry and Oral Medicine

These cysts are less important and less encountered compared to odontogenic cyst; they have no tendency to recurrence nor to neoplastic transformation.

3.2.4 Classification of Odontogenic Cysts

3.2.4.1 Nasopalatine Cyst
Also known as incisive canal cyst, this cyst typically occurs in the midline of the maxilla, associated with the nasopalatine duct. It manifests as a heart-shaped radiolucency between the central incisors, and when left untreated it can occupy all the median suture of the maxilla [12].

3.2.4.2 Stafne Cyst (Lingual Mandibular Bone Defect)
Stafne cysts are typically asymptomatic and often incidentally discovered. These lesions represent developmental anomalies, not true cysts, and appear as well-defined, corticated radiolucencies in the posterior mandible [8].

3.2.4.3 Traumatic Bone Cyst
Traumatic bone cysts are false cystic lesions that usually affect young individuals. They are called false, as they do not have the epithelial lining that normally describes true cysts. They often present as radiolucencies with well-defined borders and may be associated with a history of trauma [12].

3.2.5 Etiology and Pathogenesis

The exact etiology of these cysts remains the subject of ongoing research. Nasopalatine cysts are linked to the nasopalatine duct remnants, while Stafne cysts result from developmental defects. Traumatic bone cysts may be related to previous trauma or aseptic necrosis [8, 12, 25].

3.2.6 Clinical Presentation

Clinical signs and symptoms of these cysts are often subtle or absent. Diagnosis primarily relies on radiographic evaluations, such as panoramic radiographs, CT scans, or cone-beam computed tomography (CBCT). Biopsy and histopathological analysis are typically easy.

3.2.7 Diagnosis

After being accidently discovered, an excisional biopsy procedure normally heals the lesion [8].

3.2.8 Management and Treatment

Management of these cysts typically involves surgical enucleation to remove the lesion while preserving surrounding tissues. In the case of Stafne cysts and asymptomatic nasopalatine cysts, conservative management with observation may be considered. Postoperative complications are very rare [8, 12].

3.2.9 Complications and Their Management

Complications related to these cysts are infrequent. Prognosis is generally excellent, with low recurrence rates following surgical treatment. Long-term follow-up is typically not necessary for these lesions.

3.2.10 Conclusion

(Tip 12): In summary, nasopalatine cysts, Stafne cysts, and traumatic bone cysts are unique intraosseous lesions in the jaws. Dental and medical practitioners should be knowledgeable about their types, diagnosis, and straightforward management approaches. While these cysts may appear alarming on radiographs, their prognosis is typically favorable with appropriate treatment or observation.

3.3 Odontogenic Tumors

3.3.1 Introduction

Odontogenic tumors represent the second most common lesion in the jaws following odontogenic cyst; they are fascinating and clinically significant category of lesions that originate from the dental tissues. These tumors exhibit a remarkable range of behaviors, from benign and slow-growing to aggressive and malignant. Dentists, oral surgeons, and medical practitioners must possess a deep understanding of the various types of odontogenic tumors, their pathogenesis, and the optimal strategies for diagnosis and management [12].

3.3.2 Definition of Odontogenic Tumors

Neoplastic lesions that are derived from cells originally were part of tooth development [12].

3.3.3 Importance in Dentistry and Oral Medicine

The importance of understanding odontogenic tumors in dentistry and oral medicine cannot be underestimated. These tumors, which originate from the tissues associated with teeth, hold significant clinical relevance. Proper diagnosis and management of odontogenic tumors are crucial not only for ensuring the well-being of patients but also for preserving oral function and aesthetics. Differentiating between benign and malignant odontogenic tumors is essential, as their treatment approaches vary greatly. Furthermore, odontogenic tumors often present with symptoms that mimic other oral conditions, underscoring the necessity of a precise diagnosis. With advancements in imaging technology and molecular diagnostics, dental professionals can now provide more accurate assessments and better tailored treatment plans, ultimately improving patient outcomes and the overall quality of oral healthcare [4].

3.3.4 Classification of Odontogenic Tumors

3.3.4.1 Benign Odontogenic Tumors

Many benign odontogenic tumors can develop in the jaws. We will point at the most frequent:

1. **Ameloblastoma:** Ameloblastomas are renowned for their locally aggressive nature. Emerging from odontogenic epithelium, they often form within the mandible, although maxillary occurrences are not uncommon. The histological diversity of ameloblastomas can challenge clinicians and pathologists alike. Early detection and intervention are critical to prevent extensive tissue destruction and morbidity [12].
2. **Odontoma:** Odontomas are intriguing benign tumors characterized by the presence of dental tissues, including enamel, dentin, and sometimes cementum and pulp. These slow-growing neoplasms can resemble malformed teeth and may occasionally obstruct tooth eruption, necessitating surgical excision [12].
3. **Cementoblastoma:** Cementoblastomas are a rarity among odontogenic tumors, predominantly afflicting young individuals. These tumors arise from cementoblasts and are distinguished by their attachment to the roots of teeth. Clinical presentation often includes pain, and treatment involves the surgical extraction of the affected tooth and tumor mass [12].

3.3.4.2 Malignant Odontogenic Tumors

1. **Ameloblastic Carcinoma:** This exceedingly rare malignant tumor typically derives from ameloblastomas or arises de novo. Ameloblastic carcinomas are characterized by aggressive clinical behavior and require extensive surgical resection, often accompanied by adjuvant radiation therapy [12].

2. **Clear Cell Odontogenic Carcinoma:** Clear cell odontogenic carcinoma is an infrequent malignancy known for its distinct histological features. Effective management entails surgical excision with wide margins, and in some cases, additional adjuvant therapy may be necessary [12].
3. **Malignant Odontogenic Ghost Cell Tumor:** This tumor, linked to calcifying odontogenic cysts, displays variable clinical behavior. Surgical resection remains the primary treatment modality, although high recurrence rates necessitate diligent follow-up [12].

3.3.5 Etiology and Pathogenesis

The etiology and pathogenesis of odontogenic tumors remain subjects of intensive research. A complex interplay of genetic mutations, alterations in signaling pathways, and tissue-specific factors contribute to tumor development. For instance, mutations in the BRAF gene have been identified in some ameloblastomas, shedding light on potential therapeutic targets [12].

3.3.6 Clinical Presentation

Odontogenic tumors can manifest with a spectrum of clinical features, including pain, swelling, altered tooth eruption, or sensory disturbances like paresthesia [8, 12].

> (Tip 13): Unfortunately odontogenic tumors start developing as slow-growing silent radiolucent lesions; they are frequently underestimated as innocent odontogenic cysts and treated on this basis!

Radiographically, they frequently appear as radiolucent or mixed radiolucent-radiopaque lesions, necessitating astute clinical and radiographic examination for early recognition [8, 12].

3.3.7 Diagnosis

Accurate diagnosis hinges on comprehensive clinical evaluation, meticulous imaging studies, and, in most cases, histopathological examination. Advanced imaging modalities such as panoramic radiography, cone-beam computed tomography (CBCT), and magnetic resonance imaging (MRI) play indispensable roles in assessing tumor size, location, and invasiveness. Biopsy and histopathological analysis are indispensable for definitive diagnosis [3].

3.3.8 Management and Treatment

The management of odontogenic tumors varies considerably based on the type, extent, and potential for malignancy. Treatment options include the following:

3.3.8.1 Benign Odontogenic Tumors

1. **Surgical Excision:** Benign tumors such as odontomas are typically managed through complete surgical excision. This procedure aims to remove the tumor entirely while preserving the surrounding healthy tissue. Careful removal is essential, and postoperative follow-up is crucial to monitor for any signs of recurrence.
2. **En Bloc Resection:** Odontogenic tumors exhibiting greater aggressiveness may necessitate a more comprehensive radicular treatment strategy. Notably, conventional ameloblastomas, Pindborg tumors, and odontogenic myxomas, characterized by their heightened proclivity for recurrence, often demand en bloc resection procedures to ensure full recovery and minimize the risk of recurrence.

3.3.8.2 Malignant Odontogenic Tumors

1. **Aggressive Surgical Resection:** Malignant odontogenic tumors necessitate aggressive surgical resection with wide margins to minimize the risk of recurrence and metastasis. Surgeons may need to remove adjacent bone and soft tissues to ensure complete excision. In certain cases, adjuvant radiation therapy may be indicated to target any residual cancer cells [27].
2. **Adjuvant Treatment:** The responsibility of treating the secondary metastatic lesions of odontogenic tumors outside the oral cavity is to the oncologist; he can decide whether to apply chemotherapy, radiotherapy, or other approaches [27].

3.3.8.3 Management of Recurrent Tumor

Recurrence is a concern, particularly with ameloblastomas and certain other types of odontogenic tumors. Vigilant monitoring is imperative, and additional surgical intervention may be required if recurrence is detected. The approach to recurrent tumors may involve more extensive surgical resection and consideration of adjuvant therapies [27].

3.3.9 Complications and Their Management

Odontogenic tumors can lead to various complications, including facial deformity, functional impairment, and chronic pain. Multidisciplinary management is often necessary, involving oral and maxillofacial surgeons, oncologists, and dental specialists, to address these complications effectively [27].

3.3.10 Prognosis and Long-Term Outcomes

The prognosis for odontogenic tumors varies widely depending on factors such as tumor type, stage, and treatment efficacy. For benign tumors with complete excision, the prognosis is generally favorable, with a low risk of recurrence. Malignant odontogenic tumors have a less favorable prognosis and often require a combination of surgery and adjuvant therapies. Long-term follow-up is essential for monitoring both benign and malignant tumors [27].

3.3.11 Conclusion

(Tip 14): In summary, odontogenic tumors encompass a diverse array of lesions, ranging from benign and slow-growing tumors to aggressive malignancies. Clinicians and healthcare providers must be well-informed about the various types of odontogenic tumors, their underlying causes, and the appropriate treatment modalities. Timely diagnosis, multidisciplinary collaboration, and careful follow-up are critical to achieving the best outcomes for patients affected by odontogenic tumors.

3.4 Non-odontogenic Tumors

3.4.1 Introduction

Non-odontogenic tumors encompass a diverse group of neoplastic lesions that can develop in various regions of the body, including the head and neck. Understanding the different types, methods of diagnosis, and appropriate management strategies is crucial for medical practitioners.

3.4.2 Definition of Non-odontogenic Tumors

Neoplastic lesions that are derived from cells are not directly related to tooth development.

3.4.3 Importance in Dentistry and Oral Medicine

Non-odontogenic tumors in dentistry and oral medicine are of significant importance for several reasons:

1. **Diagnostic Challenge:** Identifying and distinguishing between odontogenic and non-odontogenic lesions can be challenging due to the overlap in clinical and radiographic features. Accurate diagnosis is crucial to determine the appropriate treatment plan.

2. **Treatment Planning:** The management of non-odontogenic tumors often varies widely from that of odontogenic tumors. An accurate diagnosis is essential for proper treatment planning, which may include surgical excision, medical management, or a combination of both.
3. **Patient Health:** Non-odontogenic tumors can affect the overall health and quality of life of patients. Some of these tumors may be benign, but others can be aggressive or even malignant, posing a risk to the patient's health and well-being.
4. **Oral Function:** Tumors in the oral cavity can impact essential functions such as speech, chewing, and swallowing. Early detection and appropriate treatment are essential to maintain these functions.
5. **Cosmetic Concerns:** Tumors in the oral and maxillofacial region can also have a significant impact on facial aesthetics. Proper management can help preserve or restore a patient's facial appearance.
6. **Interdisciplinary Collaboration:** Many non-odontogenic tumors may require collaboration with other medical specialists, such as oncologists, radiologists, and pathologists, highlighting the interdisciplinary nature of oral medicine and dentistry.
7. **Patient Education:** Dentists and oral medicine specialists play a crucial role in educating patients about the importance of regular oral examinations, which can lead to early detection and improved outcomes for non-odontogenic tumors.

> (Tip 15): Understanding and identifying non-odontogenic tumors in dentistry and oral medicine are essential for accurate diagnosis, appropriate treatment, and overall patient well-being, as they involve not only oral health but also broader medical considerations.

3.4.4 Classification of Non-odontogenic Tumors

3.4.4.1 Benign Non-odontogenic Tumors
1. **Fibro-Osseous Lesions:** Fibro-osseous lesions, including fibrous dysplasia and ossifying fibroma, can affect the jaws. They are characterized by the replacement of normal bone with fibrous tissue and varying degrees of mineralization [8, 12].
2. **Hemangioma:** Hemangiomas are benign vascular tumors that can occur in the jaws, causing localized swelling and occasional bleeding [8].
3. **Schwannoma:** Schwannomas are typically benign tumors arising from Schwann cells of the peripheral nerves. When they occur in the jaws, they often present as slow-growing, painless masses [8].

3.4.4.2 Malignant Non-odontogenic Tumors

1. **Sarcomas:** Various types of sarcomas, such as osteosarcoma and chondrosarcoma, can occur in the jaws, though they are relatively rare. These tumors are aggressive and require multidisciplinary management [8, 12].
2. **Metastatic Tumors:** Metastases from primary cancers in other parts of the body, such as breast, lung, or prostate cancer, can spread to the jaws. These metastatic lesions may present as lytic bone destruction and require careful evaluation [8].

3.4.5 Etiology and Pathogenesis

Non-odontogenic tumors in the jaws have diverse etiologies, often involving genetic mutations, environmental factors, or the abnormal growth of specific cell types. Understanding these factors is essential for effective diagnosis and management [12].

3.4.6 Clinical Presentation

1. The clinical presentation of non-odontogenic tumors in the oral and maxillofacial region can vary widely depending on the type, location, and size of the tumor. However, some common clinical features and presentations include the following [8, 13, 15, 27]:
   (a) **Swelling or Mass:** The most common presenting symptom is the presence of a painless or painful swelling or mass in the oral cavity or facial region. The size, location, and rate of growth can vary.
   (b) **Pain:** Some non-odontogenic tumors may be associated with pain, which can range from mild discomfort to severe and continuous pain.
   (c) **Ulceration:** Tumors in the oral cavity may lead to the development of ulcers on the mucosal surface, which can be painful and may bleed.
   (d) **Bleeding:** Tumors that ulcerate or erode blood vessels may result in bleeding from the oral lesion.
   (e) **Changes in Dental Occlusion:** Large tumors in the jawbones can cause changes in the alignment of teeth and bite, leading to functional problems and malocclusion.
   (f) **Neurological Symptoms:** Tumors that impinge on nerves in the head and neck region can cause sensory disturbances, such as numbness or tingling in the face.
   (g) **Difficulty in Swallowing or Speech:** Tumors located in the oral cavity or throat may interfere with swallowing or speech, leading to difficulties in these functions.

(h) **Loosening of Teeth:** Tumors in the jawbones may cause the displacement or loosening of adjacent teeth.

(i) **Facial Asymmetry:** In cases of large or rapidly growing tumors, patients may notice changes in facial appearance, resulting in facial asymmetry.

(j) **Lymphadenopathy:** Enlarged lymph nodes in the neck may be palpable if the tumor has metastasized to regional lymph nodes.

(k) **Systemic Symptoms:** In cases of malignant non-odontogenic tumors, patients may experience systemic symptoms such as weight loss, fatigue, and fever.

It's important to note that the clinical presentation can vary widely depending on the specific type of non-odontogenic tumor. Some tumors may be benign and relatively asymptomatic, while others may be aggressive or malignant, leading to more severe and rapid onset of symptoms.

Early diagnosis and appropriate medical or surgical intervention are crucial for effective management and better outcomes. Patients who experience any of these symptoms should seek prompt evaluation by a healthcare professional, ideally a dentist or oral medicine specialist, for a proper diagnosis and treatment plan.

3.4.7 Diagnosis

Accurate diagnosis relies on clinical assessment, imaging studies, and histopathological examination. Advanced imaging techniques such as CT scans, MRI, and cone-beam computed tomography (CBCT) are essential for assessing tumor size, extent, and effects on surrounding structures. Biopsy and histopathological analysis provide *definitive* diagnostic information.

3.4.8 Management and Treatment

The management of non-odontogenic tumors in the jaws depends on the specific type, extent, and potential for malignancy. Treatment options include the following [8, 12, 27]:

3.4.8.1 Benign Non-odontogenic Tumors

1. **Surgical Excision:** Benign tumors, such as fibro-osseous lesions and schwannomas, are typically managed through surgical excision. Surgeons aim to remove the tumor entirely while preserving the surrounding healthy tissue.

2. **Embolization:** In the case of hemangiomas, embolization, a minimally invasive procedure, may be employed to reduce blood flow and shrink the tumor before surgical removal.

3.4.8.2 Malignant Non-odontogenic Tumors

1. **Surgical Resection:** Malignant tumors, such as sarcomas, often require aggressive surgical resection with wide margins to minimize the risk of recurrence and spread. This may involve removal of a portion of the jawbone (resection) and, in some cases, reconstruction.
2. **Chemotherapy and Radiation:** In cases of malignant tumors, adjuvant therapies such as chemotherapy and radiation therapy may be indicated to target any residual cancer cells and improve local control.

3.4.9 Management of Recurrent Tumors

Recurrence is a concern, particularly with aggressive malignant tumors. Vigilant monitoring is imperative, and additional surgical intervention, including re-resection and adjuvant therapies, may be required if recurrence is detected.

3.4.10 Follow-Up and Monitoring

The follow-up and monitoring of non-odontogenic tumors are crucial to assess treatment outcomes, detect potential recurrences, and manage any complications. Here's a general guideline for the follow-up and monitoring of non-odontogenic tumors:

1. **Post-Treatment Evaluation:** After surgical resection or other treatments, patients should undergo an initial post-treatment evaluation to assess the surgical site, wound healing, and any immediate complications. This evaluation is typically done within the first few weeks following treatment.
2. **Histopathological Examination:** A histopathological examination of the tumor tissue is often performed to confirm the diagnosis, assess margins, and determine the tumor's characteristics. This examination provides important information for prognosis and further treatment decisions.
3. **Radiographic Follow-up:** Radiographic imaging, such as X-rays, CT scans, or MRI, is commonly used to monitor the treated area. The frequency of follow-up imaging depends on the type and stage of the tumor, but it may include regular scans for several years after treatment.
4. **Clinical Examination:** Regular clinical examinations by an oral and maxillofacial surgeon or oncologist are essential to monitor for any signs of recurrence, complications, or changes in the oral cavity or affected area. These examinations should include a thorough assessment of the surgical site and surrounding tissues.

5. **Patient Symptoms:** Patients should be encouraged to report any unusual symptoms, discomfort, or changes in the treated area promptly. Persistent pain, swelling, numbness, or other concerning symptoms should be evaluated promptly.
6. **Long-Term Follow-up:** The duration of follow-up varies depending on the tumor type and stage. Some patients may require ongoing monitoring for many years to detect late recurrences.
7. **Education and Support:** Patients should receive education about the importance of follow-up appointments and be provided with emotional support to cope with the psychological impact of cancer diagnosis and treatment.
8. **Multidisciplinary Collaboration:** In cases of malignant non-odontogenic tumors, collaboration with oncologists, radiologists, and other specialists is often necessary for comprehensive management and follow-up.
9. **Imaging Modalities:** Depending on the tumor type and clinical situation, additional imaging modalities such as PET scan (Positron Emission Tomography) or bone scans may be recommended to detect distant metastases.
10. **Biopsy or Fine-Needle Aspiration:** If there are any suspicious findings during follow-up, a biopsy or fine-needle aspiration may be performed to confirm or rule out recurrence or metastasis.
11. **Rehabilitation and Reconstruction:** For patients who have undergone extensive surgery, rehabilitation and reconstructive procedures may be part of the long-term follow-up plan to optimize function and appearance.

The follow-up and monitoring plan should be tailored to the specific characteristics of the tumor and the patient's individual risk factors. It is essential for the healthcare team to provide ongoing care, surveillance, and support to ensure the best possible outcomes for patients with non-odontogenic tumors in the oral and maxillofacial region.

3.4.11 Complications and Their Management

Non-odontogenic tumors in the jaws can lead to various complications, including facial deformity, functional impairment, and chronic pain. Multidisciplinary management is often necessary, involving oral and maxillofacial surgeons, oncologists, and dental specialists, to address these complications effectively (Fig. 3.7).

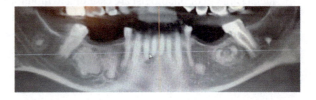

Fig. 3.7 Case of ossifying fibroma

3.4.12 Prognosis and Long-Term Outcomes

The prognosis for non-odontogenic tumors in the jaws varies widely depending on factors such as tumor type, stage, and treatment efficacy. Benign tumors generally have a favorable prognosis after complete excision. Malignant tumors require a combination of surgery and adjuvant therapies, with outcomes influenced by the tumor's aggressiveness and stage. Long-term follow-up is essential for monitoring both benign and malignant tumors.

3.4.13 Conclusion

(Tip 16): In summary, non-odontogenic tumors that affect the jaws encompass a diverse group of neoplastic conditions. Dental and medical practitioners must be well-informed about the various types of these tumors, their underlying causes, and the appropriate treatment modalities. Timely diagnosis, multidisciplinary collaboration, and careful follow-up are critical to achieving the best outcomes for patients affected by non-odontogenic tumors in the jaws.

3.5 Intraosseous Primary Malignancies

3.5.1 Introduction

Primary malignancies of the jaws are a distinct group of neoplastic conditions that originate within the bones of the maxilla and mandible. Understanding the different types, methods of diagnosis, and management strategies is crucial for dental and medical practitioners.

3.5.2 Importance in Dentistry and Oral Medicine

Intraosseous primary malignancies, also known as primary bone tumors, are tumors that originate within the bone itself, as opposed to secondary or metastatic tumors that spread to the bone from other sites in the body [8, 12]. These primary bone tumors, though relatively rare compared to other types of cancers, are important for several reasons:

1. **Early Detection and Diagnosis:** Primary bone tumors can sometimes be challenging to diagnose because their symptoms, such as pain and swelling, may mimic other more common conditions. However, early detection is crucial for better treatment outcomes. Dentists, orthopedic surgeons, and other healthcare

professionals who are knowledgeable about primary bone tumors play a critical role in recognizing and diagnosing these conditions.

2. **Treatment Planning:** Accurate diagnosis of intraosseous primary malignancies is essential for determining the most appropriate treatment strategy. Treatment options can include surgery, radiation therapy, chemotherapy, or a combination of these modalities. The type and extent of treatment depend on the specific tumor type, stage, and location within the bone.

3. **Prognosis:** The prognosis for patients with intraosseous primary malignancies varies widely based on factors such as tumor type, size, location, and stage at diagnosis. Some primary bone tumors have a relatively good prognosis when detected early and treated appropriately, while others may be more aggressive. Understanding the tumor's characteristics is vital for providing patients with accurate information about their prognosis.

4. **Quality of Life:** Bone tumors can significantly impact a patient's quality of life by causing pain, functional limitations, and deformities. Proper management and treatment of these tumors aim to alleviate symptoms and improve the patient's quality of life.

5. **Research and Advances in Treatment:** Studying primary bone tumors can lead to advances in cancer research and treatment strategies. Insights gained from primary bone tumor research can contribute to a broader understanding of cancer biology, which may benefit patients with other types of malignancies.

6. **Multidisciplinary Care:** The management of primary bone tumors often requires a multidisciplinary approach involving head and neck surgeons, oncologists, radiologists, oral maxillofacial pathologists, and other healthcare professionals. Collaboration among these specialists is crucial for optimizing patient care and treatment outcomes.

7. **Patient Awareness:** Raising awareness about primary bone tumors and their symptoms is essential for encouraging individuals to seek medical attention when experiencing concerning signs. Early diagnosis and intervention can lead to better outcomes and improved survival rates.

(Tip 17): Primary bone tumors, while relatively rare, are important in the fields of medicine and oncology because of their potential impact on patients' lives, the need for accurate diagnosis and treatment planning, and their contribution to cancer research and treatment advancements. Healthcare professionals play a pivotal role in recognizing and managing these tumors to provide the best possible care for affected individuals.

3.5.3 Classification of Primary Intraosseous Malignancies

3.5.3.1 Primary Bone Sarcomas

1. **Osteosarcoma:** Osteosarcoma is the most common primary malignant bone tumor in the jaws. It is characterized by the production of osteoid or immature bone by tumor cells. These tumors often manifest as painful, rapidly growing masses [12].
2. **Chondrosarcoma:** Chondrosarcomas in the jaws arise from cartilage-forming cells within the bone. They can affect various parts of the jaws, leading to pain and swelling [12].
3. **Ewing Sarcoma:** Ewing sarcoma is a rare but highly aggressive malignancy that primarily affects children and young adults. It usually arises in the bones of the jaw, causing significant morbidity [8].

3.5.3.2 Other Primary Jaw Tumors

1. **Ameloblastic Carcinoma:** While ameloblastomas are typically benign, ameloblastic carcinomas are malignant transformations of these tumors. They can occur in the jaws and require aggressive management [12].
2. **Mucoepidermoid Carcinoma:** Mucoepidermoid carcinomas are malignant salivary gland tumors that may involve the jawbones, particularly the mandible. They can present as painless swellings [12].
3. **Intraosseous Squamous Cell Carcinoma:** Ontraosseous or central sqouamous cell carcinoma are extremely rare, still up-to 100 cases in the literature have been reported [1, 8].

3.5.4 Etiology and Pathogenesis

Intraosseous primary malignancies in the jaws, also known as primary jaw bone tumors or primary oral malignancies, have a complex etiology and pathogenesis influenced by various factors. These tumors can arise within the maxilla (upper jaw) or mandible (lower jaw) and may include several histological types. The exact cause of these tumors is not always well-understood, but several factors may contribute to their development:

1. **Genetic Factors:** Genetic mutations and alterations in DNA can play a role in the development of intraosseous jaw tumors. Some individuals may inherit genetic predispositions that increase their susceptibility to certain malignancies, while others may acquire genetic mutations during their lifetime [12].
2. **Environmental Factors:** Exposure to carcinogens and environmental toxins can contribute to the development of oral malignancies. Smoking and tobacco use, alcohol consumption, and exposure to ionizing radiation are known risk factors for intraosseous jaw tumors [28].
3. **Viral Infections:** Some studies have suggested a potential link between certain viral infections and the development of jaw tumors. For example, the human

papillomavirus (HPV) has been associated with an increased risk of oral squamous cell carcinoma, which can occur in the jaws [29].

4. **Chronic Irritation and Trauma:** Chronic irritation or trauma to the oral mucosa or jawbones can create an environment conducive to the development of malignancies. Repeated injury or irritation may lead to inflammation and cell damage, increasing the risk of malignant transformation [12].
5. **Pre-existing Conditions:** Certain pre-existing oral conditions, such as conditions associated with chronic inflammation, may increase the risk of malignancy in the jawbones [12].
6. **Radiation Exposure:** Previous exposure to radiation therapy in the head and neck region for other medical conditions can elevate the risk of developing primary jaw tumors, particularly osteosarcomas [12].
7. **Genetic Syndromes:** Some genetic syndromes, such as Li-Fraumeni syndrome and hereditary retinoblastoma, are associated with an increased risk of developing primary bone tumors in the jaws [12].

The pathogenesis of intraosseous primary malignancies in the jaws involves a multistep process that includes initiation, promotion, and progression [30]:

1. **Initiation:** Genetic mutations or alterations in specific genes may initiate the transformation of normal cells into cancerous cells within the jawbone. These mutations may be caused by factors like genetic predisposition, environmental exposures, or viral infections.
2. **Promotion:** Once initiated, the cancerous cells undergo further changes that promote their growth and proliferation. This stage can be influenced by factors such as chronic inflammation, carcinogens, or genetic mutations.
3. **Progression:** Progression involves the continued growth and invasion of cancer cells into surrounding tissues, leading to the development of a clinically detectable tumor. The specific characteristics and behavior of the tumor depend on its histological type.

Early detection and diagnosis are critical in improving the prognosis of intraosseous primary malignancies in the jaws. Treatment typically involves surgical resection, radiation therapy, and, in some cases, chemotherapy. Multidisciplinary collaboration among head and neck surgeons, oncologists, radiologists, and oral and maxillofacial pathologists is essential for effective management and care of patients with these malignancies.

3.5.5 Clinical Presentation

Intraosseous primary malignancies in the jaws can present with a range of clinical signs and symptoms. The specific presentation may vary depending on the type and stage of the malignancy, but here are some common clinical features [8]:

1. **Pain:** Persistent and often severe pain is a frequent symptom. It may be localized to the jaw area and can sometimes radiate to the ear or adjacent facial

regions. Pain is often a key indicator that prompts individuals to seek medical attention.

2. **Swelling and Facial Asymmetry:** A noticeable swelling or lump in the jaw region is a common finding. This swelling may cause facial asymmetry and may be accompanied by tenderness or warmth in the affected area.

3. **Loose Teeth:** In cases where the tumor affects the supporting bone, individuals may experience loosening of teeth or a change in dental alignment and occlusion.

4. **Paresthesia:** Numbness or tingling sensations in the lips, chin, or other facial areas can occur when the tumor impinges on nerves within the jawbone.

5. **Ulceration or Mucosal Changes:** Malignant lesions in the jaw may cause ulceration of the overlying oral mucosa, resulting in open sores that do not heal. These ulcers can be painful and may bleed.

6. **Difficulty in Chewing or Speaking:** As the tumor grows, it can interfere with normal oral function, leading to difficulties in chewing, swallowing, or speaking.

7. **Dental Mobility:** Mobility of teeth in the vicinity of the tumor may be observed due to the destruction of supporting bone.

8. **Palpable Lymph Nodes:** If the malignancy has spread to regional lymph nodes, palpable lymph node enlargement in the neck may be detected during a physical examination.

9. **Unexplained Weight Loss:** Some individuals may experience unexplained weight loss, fatigue, or malaise, which can be associated with advanced malignancies.

10. **Visible or Radiographic Lesions:** Dental or medical professionals may detect visible lesions during a routine oral examination, or they may observe abnormalities on radiographic images (X-rays, CT scans, or MRI scans) taken for other reasons.

11. **Altered Bite or Facial Deformity:** Advanced intraosseous jaw tumors can cause significant changes in bite alignment and facial contour, leading to noticeable deformities.

It is essential to note that the clinical presentation of intraosseous primary malignancies can mimic other non-malignant conditions, such as dental infections or benign tumors. However, any persistent, unexplained symptoms in the jaw, especially pain, swelling, or mobility of teeth, should be promptly evaluated by a healthcare professional.

Early diagnosis is crucial for timely treatment and improved outcomes for patients with primary jaw bone malignancies. The diagnosis is typically confirmed through a combination of clinical evaluation, imaging studies, and, on top, biopsy and histopathological examination of the tissue.

3.5.6 Differential Diagnosis

Consider the following primary malignancies in the jaws [8, 12]:

1. **Osteosarcoma:** A malignant bone tumor, typically found in adolescents and young adults.
2. **Chondrosarcoma:** Arises from cartilaginous tissue within the jaw.
3. **Ameloblastic Carcinoma:** A malignant transformation of ameloblastoma, a benign odontogenic tumor.
4. **Adenoid Cystic Carcinoma:** Another salivary gland tumor that may affect the jaws.
5. **Mucoepidermoid Carcinoma:** A salivary gland malignancy that can involve the jaw as a primary centric malignancy.
6. **Ewing's Sarcoma:** Rare but can occur in the jawbones.
7. **Central Squamous Cell Carcinoma:** Most common primary malignancy in the oral cavity, often arising from the oral mucosa. Rare cases have been reported intraosseous.

3.5.7 Diagnosis

Accurate diagnosis of primary malignancies in the jaws relies on clinical assessment, advanced imaging studies, and histopathological examination. Radiographic techniques like CT scans and MRI are essential for assessing tumor size, extent, and effects on surrounding structures. Biopsy and histopathological analysis provide definitive diagnostic information.

The guideline should be as follows:

1. **Clinical Presentation:**
   Start by gathering information about the patient's symptoms, including pain, swelling, numbness, or changes in dentition.
   Note the location and extent of the lesion within the jaw.
2. **Medical History:**
   Obtain the patient's medical history, including any history of cancer, radiation therapy, or chemotherapy.
   Assess for any systemic conditions that may contribute to jaw lesions (e.g., Paget's disease).
3. **Radiographic Evaluation:**
   Conduct imaging studies such as panoramic radiographs, CT scans, or MRI to assess the lesion's size, shape, and relationship to adjacent structures.
   Evaluate for bone destruction, sclerosis, or periosteal reaction.
4. **Histopathological Examination:**
   Tissue biopsy is essential for definitive diagnosis. Perform an incisional or excisional biopsy as indicated.
   Send the biopsy specimen for histopathological analysis to determine the type of tumor.

3.5.8 Management and Treatment

The management of primary malignancies in the jaws is complex and varies depending on the specific type, stage, and location of the tumor. Treatment options include the following [8, 27]:

3.5.8.1 Primary Bone Sarcomas
1. **Surgical Resection:** Surgical removal is often the primary treatment for osteosarcoma, chondrosarcoma, and Ewing sarcoma. Surgeons aim to remove the tumor with wide margins while preserving function and minimizing complications. Reconstruction may be necessary, particularly in cases of extensive resection.
2. **Chemotherapy:** Neoadjuvant and adjuvant chemotherapy are often employed in conjunction with surgery for osteosarcoma and Ewing sarcoma to target micrometastases and improve local control.
3. **Radiation Therapy:** Radiation therapy may be used in select cases, such as unresectable tumors or when limb-sparing surgery is not feasible. However, it is less commonly utilized in primary bone sarcomas of the jaws compared to soft tissue sarcomas due to potential adverse effects on bone healing.

3.5.8.2 Other Primary Jaw Tumors
1. **Ameloblastic Carcinoma:** Surgical resection with wide margins is the mainstay of treatment for ameloblastic carcinoma. Adjuvant radiation therapy may be considered in some cases.
2. **Mucoepidermoid Carcinoma:** Treatment of mucoepidermoid carcinoma may involve surgical resection with consideration of adjuvant therapies such as radiation.

3.5.9 Management of Recurrent Malignancies

Recurrence is a concern in primary malignancies of the jaws, particularly in cases of aggressive tumors. Vigilant monitoring and additional treatment, including re-resection, radiation therapy, or systemic therapies, may be necessary if recurrence occurs (Fig. 3.8).

3.5.10 Complications and Their Management

Primary malignancies in the jaws can lead to complications such as pain, infection, facial deformity, and functional impairment. A multidisciplinary team of healthcare professionals, including oral and maxillofacial surgeons, oncologists, and rehabilitation specialists, is often required to manage these complications effectively.

Here's an overview of some common complications and their management [31]:

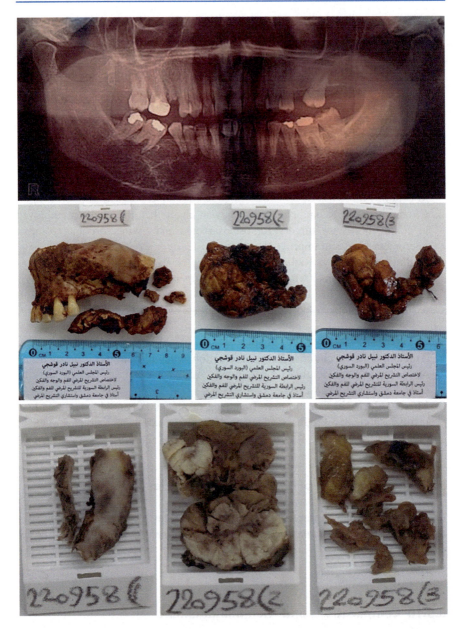

Fig. 3.8 Fibrosarcoma detailed case. This poor lady, 52 years old, suffered from fibrosarcoma, the late diagnosis was mainly due to thoughts that it can be an odontogenic tumor, and there is no need to further evaluation; after final diagnosis was established, cervical nodule involvement was discovered, and neck dissection operation was performed

3.5.10.1 Local Invasion

Complication: Malignant tumors can invade adjacent structures such as teeth, nerves, blood vessels, and sinuses.

Management: Complete surgical resection with clear margins is the primary treatment to prevent local recurrence. In some cases, reconstruction of affected structures may be necessary.

3.5.10.2 Pathological Fractures

Complication: Malignant tumors weaken the jawbone, making it susceptible to fractures.

Management: Stabilization of the fractured jawbone through surgery, often with the use of plates, screws, or bone grafts, followed by treatment of the underlying malignancy.

3.5.10.3 Pain and Discomfort

Complication: Patients may experience pain and discomfort due to tumor growth and tissue destruction.

Management: Pain management strategies may include analgesics, opioids, non-steroidal anti-inflammatory drugs (NSAIDs), and palliative care for advanced cases.

3.5.10.4 Swelling and Facial Deformity

Complication: Tumor growth can cause noticeable facial swelling and deformity.

Management: Surgical resection, reconstruction, and orthognathic surgery to restore facial aesthetics and function.

3.5.10.5 Trismus (Limited Mouth Opening)

Complication: Tumors in the jaw can restrict mouth opening.

Management: Physical therapy and jaw exercises to improve mouth opening. In some cases, surgical release of fibrous bands (myotomy) may be required.

3.5.10.6 Nerve Damage

Complication: Nerves in the jaw region may be compressed or invaded by tumors, leading to sensory or motor deficits.

Management: Nerve-sparing surgical techniques may be used whenever possible. Rehabilitation and therapy to improve nerve function after treatment.

3.5.10.7 Osteoradionecrosis (ORN)

Complication: Radiation therapy can damage the jawbone, leading to the development of non-healing ulcers or exposed bone.

Management: Hyperbaric oxygen therapy, antibiotics, and surgical debridement for severe cases. Prevention strategies include proper dental care before radiation therapy.

3.5.10.8 Hemorrhage

Complication: Tumor-related vascularization may lead to bleeding.

Management: Control bleeding during surgery, and consider preoperative embolization in highly vascular tumors.

3.5.10.9 Metastasis

Complication: Spread of malignancy to distant sites.

Management: Monitoring for metastasis through imaging and regular follow-up. Treatment with systemic therapies (chemotherapy, immunotherapy) when appropriate.

3.5.10.10 Psychological and Quality of Life Issues

Complication: Patients and their families may experience psychological distress due to the diagnosis and treatment.

Management: Offer psychological support, counseling, and palliative care services to improve quality of life.

> (Tip 18): Management of complications in intraosseous malignancies of the jaws requires a multidisciplinary approach involving oral and maxillofacial surgeons, oncologists, radiation oncologists, dental specialists, and other healthcare professionals. The choice of management depends on the specific nature of the malignancy, its stage, and the overall health of the patient.

3.5.11 Prognosis and Long-Term Outcomes

The prognosis for patients with primary malignancies in the jaws varies widely depending on factors such as tumor type, stage, and treatment response. Early diagnosis and multimodal treatment approaches are essential for achieving the best outcomes. Long-term follow-up is crucial for monitoring patients for recurrence and late effects of treatment.

3.5.11.1 Variety of Tumor Types

Malignancies of the intraosseous of the jaws can include various types of tumors, such as odontogenic carcinomas, osteosarcomas, and chondrosarcomas. Prognosis varies significantly based on the specific type.

3.5.11.2 Prognostic Factors

Several factors influence prognosis:

- **Histological Grade:** Tumor grade (low, intermediate, high) is a significant predictor of outcomes. High-grade tumors tend to have worse prognoses.
- **Tumor Size:** Larger tumors are generally associated with poorer outcomes.
- **Metastasis:** The presence of distant metastasis (spread to other parts of the body) significantly worsens prognosis.

- **Early Detection:** Early diagnosis and intervention are crucial for better outcomes. Routine dental check-ups and imaging can aid in early detection.
- **Treatment Modalities:** Treatment usually involves surgery, which may include resection of the tumor and reconstruction with bone grafts or other materials. Radiation therapy and chemotherapy may be necessary depending on the tumor type and stage.
- **Recurrence:** Some intraosseous jaw malignancies have a tendency to recur. Regular follow-up and imaging are essential to monitor for recurrence.
- **Functional Outcomes:** The location and extent of the tumor can affect jaw function and facial appearance. Reconstructive surgery aims to restore both form and function.
- **Quality of Life:** Survivors of jaw malignancies often face challenges related to eating, speech, and appearance. Support from dental professionals and multidisciplinary teams can improve the quality of life.
- **Survival Rates:** Survival rates vary widely depending on the specific tumor type, stage at diagnosis, and treatment.
- **Patient Education:** It's important to educate patients about the potential long-term effects of treatment, such as dental issues, jaw function, and psychosocial aspects.
- **Emotional Support:** Patients and their families may benefit from counseling and support groups to cope with the emotional and psychological challenges of dealing with jaw malignancies.
- **Research and Advancements:** Ongoing research and advancements in cancer treatment may lead to improved outcomes in the future. Encourage patients to stay informed about potential treatment options.
- **Multidisciplinary Care:** Collaboration between oral and maxillofacial surgeons, oncologists, radiologists, and dental specialists is critical for comprehensive care and achieving the best possible outcomes.

> (Tip 19): Please note that specific prognosis and long-term outcomes can vary widely depending on individual cases and the precise characteristics of the tumor. It's essential for patients to consult with healthcare professionals for personalized information and guidance regarding their condition.

3.5.12 Conclusion

> (Tip 20): In summary, primary malignancies of the jaws encompass a unique group of neoplastic conditions that require specialized knowledge and management. Dental and medical practitioners must be well-informed about the different types of these tumors, their etiology, and the appropriate treatment modalities. Timely diagnosis, multidisciplinary collaboration, and vigilant follow-up are essential for achieving the best outcomes for patients affected by primary malignancies in the jaws.

3.6 Intraosseous Secondary (Metastatic) Malignancies

3.6.1 Introduction

Metastatic malignancies affecting the jaws represent a unique and clinically significant category of neoplastic conditions. These tumors originate in distant organs and tissues before spreading to the jawbones. Understanding the various types, diagnostic approaches, and management strategies is essential for dental and medical practitioners.

3.6.2 Importance in Dentistry and Oral Medicine

Certainly, intraosseous secondary (metastatic) malignancies in the jaws, which occur within the bone of the jaw rather than in the soft tissues of the mouth, are important in dentistry for several reasons [32].

3.6.2.1 Early Detection
Dentists often play a crucial role in the early detection of these secondary malignancies. Routine dental check-ups and radiographic imaging (such as dental X-rays and panoramic radiographs) can reveal abnormalities or lesions in the jawbones. The early identification of metastatic lesions can lead to prompt diagnosis and treatment.

3.6.2.2 Differential Diagnosis
Dentists must differentiate between benign and malignant lesions in the jawbones. Secondary malignancies in the jaws may mimic benign conditions or cysts, making accurate diagnosis challenging. Dentists with expertise in oral maxillofacial pathology can help distinguish between various pathologies and refer patients to specialists for further evaluation if necessary.

3.6.2.3 Treatment Planning
Once metastatic malignancies are identified, dentists collaborate with oncologists and other healthcare professionals to plan comprehensive treatment. This may involve surgical resection, radiation therapy, chemotherapy, or a combination of these treatments. Dental health and function are essential considerations in treatment planning, as surgery and radiation can affect oral and dental structures.

3.6.2.4 Oral Health Maintenance
Patients with metastatic malignancies in the jaws often require specialized dental care to manage potential complications. This includes addressing dental infections, ensuring proper oral hygiene, and managing dental and oral side effects of cancer treatments. Dentists help maintain the oral health and comfort of these patients throughout their cancer journey [32].

3.6.2.5 Reconstruction and Prosthodontics

In cases where surgical resection is necessary, dentists and prosthodontists are involved in reconstructing and restoring the jaws and dentition. This may include the placement of dental implants, removable prostheses, or other interventions to improve oral function and appearance post-treatment.

3.6.2.6 Pain and Symptom Management

Metastatic malignancies in the jaws can cause significant pain and discomfort. Dentists can assist in managing oral pain and symptoms, helping patients maintain a reasonable quality of life during their cancer treatment.

3.6.2.7 Multidisciplinary Collaboration

Dentists work closely with oncologists, oral and maxillofacial surgeons, radiologists, and other healthcare providers to ensure comprehensive care for patients with metastatic jaw malignancies. Multidisciplinary collaboration is essential to address all aspects of the disease and its impact on oral health.

3.6.2.8 Psychosocial Support

Dentists also provide emotional support and guidance to patients and their families. A cancer diagnosis can be emotionally challenging, and dentists can help patients navigate the dental aspects of their treatment while offering reassurance and empathy.

(Tip 21): In summary, the importance of intraosseous secondary malignancies in the jaws in dentistry lies in their early detection, accurate diagnosis, comprehensive treatment planning, and ongoing oral health management. Dentists play a vital role in the multidisciplinary care team, ensuring that patients receive the best possible dental care in the context of their cancer treatment.

3.6.3 Classification of Primary Malignancies

3.6.3.1 Common Primary Sites for Jaw Metastases [8, 15]

1. **Breast Cancer:** Breast cancer is one of the most common sources of metastases to the jaws. These tumors often manifest as lytic lesions in the mandible and maxilla [33].
2. **Lung Cancer:** Lung cancer can metastasize to the jaws, presenting with similar radiographic features as other primary sources. Diagnosis involves imaging and, in some cases, biopsy [33].
3. **Renal Cell Carcinoma:** Renal cell carcinoma is known for its propensity to metastasize to various organs, including the jaws. These metastases can be expansile and destructive [33].

3.6.3.2 Other Primary Sites

1. **Prostate Cancer:** Prostate cancer can rarely metastasize to the jaws. While uncommon, it can lead to significant jawbone involvement.
2. **Thyroid Cancer:** Papillary thyroid carcinoma may metastasize to the jaws. These metastases may resemble other benign jaw lesions, necessitating histopathological evaluation for definitive diagnosis.

3.6.4 Etiology and Pathogenesis

Metastatic malignancies in the jaws occur when cancer cells from a primary tumor site enter the bloodstream or lymphatic system, disseminate to the jaws, and establish secondary tumors. Understanding the mechanisms behind this process is essential for effective management.

> (Tip 22): The etiology (causes) and pathogenesis (development) of intraosseous secondary (metastatic) malignancies in the jaws are rooted in the spread of cancer from primary sites elsewhere in the body to the jawbones.

Here are the key points regarding their etiology and pathogenesis [33]:

3.6.4.1 Etiology

Metastasis from Primary Cancer: Intraosseous secondary malignancies in the jaws occur when cancer cells from a primary tumor located elsewhere in the body (e.g., breast, lung, prostate, kidney) spread or metastasize to the jawbones. This is the primary cause of secondary jaw malignancies [33].

Hematogenous/lymphogenous Spread: Cancer cells typically reach the jaws through the bloodstream (hematogenous spread) or lymphatic vessels. They travel from the primary tumor site to the jawbones via vessels, where they can establish secondary tumor growth [33].

Tumor Cell Characteristics: Certain types of cancer have a greater tendency to metastasize to the jaws. For example, breast and lung cancers are more commonly associated with metastases to the jawbones [33].

Site of Metastasis: The specific location within the jaw where metastatic tumors develop can vary. They may occur in the mandible or the maxilla, and their distribution can influence clinical presentation [32].

3.6.4.2 Pathogenesis

Microenvironment: The development of secondary jaw malignancies is influenced by the microenvironment of the jawbones. Bone tissue provides a fertile ground for cancer cells to implant and grow due to its rich blood supply and availability of growth factors.

Invasion and Colonization: Cancer cells from the primary tumor site invade nearby blood vessels, allowing them to enter the bloodstream. Once in circulation, they can travel to distant sites, including the jaws. Cancer cells adhere to the vascular endothelium in the jaw, escape the bloodstream, and then proliferate within the bone tissue.

Formation of Metastatic Tumor: Once cancer cells establish themselves in the jawbone, they begin to form a secondary tumor. This process involves rapid cell division and angiogenesis (formation of new blood vessels) to supply the growing tumor with nutrients and oxygen.

> (Tip 23): It's important to note that the etiology and pathogenesis of secondary jaw malignancies are primarily related to the behavior of the primary cancer and its ability to spread to distant sites. Early detection, accurate diagnosis, and appropriate treatment are essential to manage these metastatic lesions effectively.

3.6.5 Clinical Presentation

Jaws metastatic malignancies may present with various clinical features, including pain, swelling, tooth mobility, or pathologic fractures. Dental and medical practitioners should consider metastatic malignancies in the differential diagnosis of jaw lesions, particularly in patients with a history of cancer. The specific symptoms depend on the location and size of the secondary tumor.

The clinical presentation of intraosseous secondary (metastatic) malignancies in the jaws can vary depending on several factors, including the site of the metastasis, the size of the tumor, the type of cancer involved, and the individual patient's response. Here are some common clinical presentations and symptoms associated with these secondary jaw malignancies [8, 15]:

1. **Localized Pain:** One of the most common symptoms is localized pain in the affected jaw area. This pain can be persistent, progressive, and may worsen over time. It is often described as a dull, aching sensation.
2. **Swelling:** Patients may notice swelling or enlargement of the jaw, which can be palpable (able to be felt) or visible. Swelling may be accompanied by tenderness to touch.
3. **Oral Dysfunction:** Depending on the location and size of the metastatic tumor, patients may experience changes in oral function. This can include difficulty chewing, speaking, or swallowing. Large tumors can impact the alignment of the teeth or interfere with dentures.
4. **Paresthesia:** Paresthesia refers to abnormal sensations such as numbness, tingling, or altered sensation in the jaw, lips, or chin. This can occur when the tumor presses on or infiltrates nearby nerves.

5. **Tooth Mobility:** In some cases, the metastatic tumor can cause tooth mobility or looseness due to its effect on the surrounding bone and supporting structures.
6. **Pathological Fracture:** Advanced secondary jaw malignancies can weaken the jawbone to the point where it becomes susceptible to pathological fractures. Patients may experience a sudden fracture of the jawbone without significant trauma.
7. **Ulceration or Erosion of the Oral Mucosa:** Depending on the location of the tumor, it may cause ulceration or erosion of the overlying oral mucosa (the lining of the mouth). This can lead to pain and discomfort.
8. **Facial Asymmetry:** In cases where the tumor causes significant jawbone enlargement, patients may notice facial asymmetry or changes in their facial appearance.
9. **General Systemic Symptoms:** In some instances, patients with metastatic jaw malignancies may experience systemic symptoms, such as weight loss, fatigue, and a decline in overall health. These symptoms are often associated with advanced disease.
10. **Spontaneous Bleeding:** In rare cases, metastatic tumors in the jaws may lead to spontaneous bleeding or ulceration of the oral mucosa.

(Tip 24): It's important to emphasize that the clinical presentation can vary widely, and not all patients will experience the same symptoms. Additionally, some individuals may remain asymptomatic until the tumor has reached an advanced stage. Because of this variability, it's crucial for individuals to seek prompt evaluation by a healthcare provider if they notice any unusual or persistent symptoms related to their jaw or oral health. Early detection and diagnosis are essential for effective management and treatment of metastatic jaw malignancies.

3.6.6 Diagnosis

Accurate diagnosis of jaws metastatic malignancies relies on clinical evaluation, imaging studies, and histopathological examination. Advanced imaging modalities such as CT scans, MRI, and PET scans are valuable for assessing the extent and distribution of metastases. Biopsy and histopathological analysis are essential for definitive diagnosis.

The diagnosis of intraosseous secondary (metastatic) malignancies in the jaws involves a series of steps, including clinical evaluation, imaging studies, and histopathological examination. Additionally, a differential diagnosis is essential to distinguish these malignancies from other benign and malignant conditions that can affect the jaws. Here's an overview of the diagnostic process and the differential diagnosis:

3.6.6.1 Diagnostic Process

1. **Clinical Evaluation:** The diagnostic process often begins with a thorough clinical examination by a dentist, oral and maxillofacial surgeon, or an oral medicine specialist. The healthcare provider will assess the patient's medical history and perform a physical examination of the oral and maxillofacial region. They will look for signs and symptoms such as pain, swelling, changes in oral function, and any other abnormalities.

2. **Imaging Studies:**
   Diagnostic Imaging: Radiographic imaging, such as dental X-rays and CT scans, is often used to detect these lesions. Radiologists and oral and maxillofacial specialists evaluate the characteristics of the tumor to determine its origin and extent.
   (a) Radiography: Dental X-rays, panoramic radiographs, and cone-beam computed tomography (CBCT) scans are commonly used to visualize the jawbone and any lesions within it. These imaging modalities can help identify the presence of a lesion and its characteristics.
   (b) Computed tomography (CT) or magnetic resonance imaging (MRI): For more detailed information and to assess the extent of the lesion, a CT or MRI scan may be ordered. These imaging techniques provide cross-sectional views and can help determine if the lesion has infiltrated nearby structures.

3. **Biopsy:**
   A definitive diagnosis of a jaw malignancy requires a tissue biopsy. A small sample of the lesion is taken through a minimally invasive procedure, often performed by an oral surgeon or oral maxillofcial pathologist. The biopsy is sent to a pathology laboratory for histological examination.

4. **Histopathological Examination:** Pathologists examine the biopsy specimen under a microscope to determine the type of cells present, their characteristics, and whether they are indicative of malignancy. This step is crucial in confirming the diagnosis. This information helps guide treatment planning.

3.6.6.2 Differential Diagnosis

In diagnosing intraosseous secondary malignancies in the jaws, it is important to consider and rule out other conditions that can mimic similar clinical and radiographic features. The following are some of the conditions that may be included in the differential diagnosis:

1. **Benign Jaw Lesions:**
   (a) Odontogenic cysts (e.g., radicular cyst, dentigerous cyst).
   (b) Benign tumors (e.g., ameloblastoma, osteoma).
   (c) Fibro-osseous lesions (e.g., fibrous dysplasia).
2. **Other Malignant Lesions:**
   (a) Primary jaw malignancies (e.g., osteosarcoma, chondrosarcoma).
   (b) Lymphomas involving the jawbone.
   (c) Metastatic lesions from primary cancers at other head and neck sites.

3. **Infectious Conditions:**
   (a) Chronic osteomyelitis or osteonecrosis of the jaw.
   (b) Inflammatory conditions.
   (c) Sarcoidosis or other granulomatous diseases involving the jaws.
4. **Vascular Lesions:**
   (a) Vascular malformations that may appear as radiolucent areas on imaging.
5. **Dental Lesions:**
   (a) Periapical granulomas or cysts.
   (b) Residual dental socket after tooth extraction.

To differentiate between these conditions, clinicians rely on a combination of clinical findings, radiographic features, and histopathological examination. The specific characteristics of the lesion on imaging and the cellular features seen under the microscope can help establish a definitive diagnosis and guide treatment planning.

> (Tip 25): Ultimately, a multidisciplinary approach involving oral and maxillofacial surgeons, pathologists, radiologists, and oncologists is often required to arrive at an accurate diagnosis and develop an appropriate treatment plan for intraosseous secondary jaw malignancies.

3.6.7 Management and Treatment

The management of jaws metastatic malignancies primarily focuses on palliation and improving the patient's quality of life. Treatment options include the following:

1. **Pain Management:** Effective pain management is a key aspect of care. This may involve medications such as opioids and non-steroidal anti-inflammatory drugs (NSAIDs), as well as non-pharmacological interventions like radiation therapy.
2. **Radiation Therapy:** Radiation therapy is often used to alleviate pain and reduce tumor size in jaws metastatic malignancies. It can provide relief and improve oral function.
3. **Surgical Intervention:** Surgery may be considered for select cases, such as pathologic fractures or when tumors impede essential functions like swallowing or breathing. Surgical procedures aim to enhance quality of life and may involve tumor debulking or stabilization.

3.6.8 Management of Recurrent Malignancies

Recurrence is a concern in metastatic malignancies, particularly when cancer is aggressive. Vigilant monitoring and ongoing management are crucial to address recurrent metastases.

Managing recurrent malignancies in the jaws, whether primary or secondary (metastatic), is a complex and challenging process that requires a multidisciplinary approach. The management of recurrent malignancies involves several key considerations:

1. **Accurate Diagnosis:**
   Before initiating any treatment for recurrent malignancies, it's essential to confirm the diagnosis through biopsy and pathological examination. This helps determine the type of cancer, its grade, and other critical factors that influence treatment decisions.
2. **Multidisciplinary Team:**
   A multidisciplinary team of healthcare professionals, including oral and maxillofacial surgeons, oncologists, radiation oncologists, medical oncologists, and radiologists, should collaborate to develop an individualized treatment plan.
3. **Treatment Options:**
   The choice of treatment for recurrent malignancies depends on various factors, including the type of cancer, the location and size of the recurrence, the patient's overall health, and previous treatments. Common treatment options include the following:
   Surgery: Surgical resection of the recurrent tumor may be considered if it is localized and resectable. This can involve wide excision and reconstruction.
   Radiation Therapy: Radiation therapy may be used either alone or in combination with surgery to treat recurrent tumors. It can be delivered externally (external beam radiation) or internally (brachytherapy).
   Chemotherapy: Systemic chemotherapy may be used to treat recurrent malignancies, especially if they are widespread or have metastasized to other parts of the body.
   Targeted Therapies: In some cases, targeted therapies that focus on specific molecular pathways associated with the cancer may be recommended.
   Immunotherapy: Immunotherapies that enhance the body's immune response against cancer cells are being explored as potential treatments for recurrent malignancies.
4. **Palliative Care:**
   In cases where recurrent malignancies are advanced and treatment options are limited, palliative care becomes a crucial component of management.

> (Tip 26): Palliative care focuses on relieving symptoms, improving the patient's quality of life, and providing emotional and psychological support.

5. **Rehabilitation and Reconstruction:**
   Recurrent malignancies, especially those that require surgical resection, can result in significant functional and aesthetic deficits. Rehabilitation and reconstructive procedures are often necessary to restore oral function and appearance. This may involve dental implants, bone grafts, or prosthetic devices.

6. **Surveillance and Follow-up:**

    After treatment, patients with recurrent malignancies require vigilant surveillance and regular follow-up appointments. Imaging studies and clinical assessments are used to monitor for any signs of disease recurrence.

7. **Supportive Care:**

    Patients dealing with recurrent malignancies benefit from supportive care services such as pain management, nutritional support, and psychosocial support. Support groups and counseling can help address the emotional and psychological aspects of cancer recurrence.

8. **Clinical Trials:**

    Participation in clinical trials may be an option for some patients with recurrent malignancies. These trials offer access to experimental treatments and therapies that are not yet widely available.

> (Tip 27): It's important to note that the management of recurrent malignancies is highly individualized. Treatment decisions are influenced by the specific characteristics of the recurrence, the patient's overall health, and their preferences. The goal of management is to achieve the best possible outcomes while addressing the unique challenges associated with recurrent jaw malignancies. Open and ongoing communication between the patient and the healthcare team is essential throughout the treatment process.

3.6.9 Follow-Up and Monitoring

Follow-up and monitoring are crucial aspects of the care for patients who have been treated for intraosseous secondary (metastatic) malignancies in the jaws or any other form of jaw malignancy.

The purpose of follow-up and monitoring is to:

1. **Detect Recurrence:** Regular follow-up appointments and monitoring are essential to detect any signs of cancer recurrence as early as possible. Early detection can lead to more effective treatment options.
2. **Evaluate Treatment Response:** Monitoring allows healthcare providers to assess how well the patient is responding to treatment. This information can guide adjustments to the treatment plan if necessary.
3. **Manage Treatment-Related Side Effects:** Patients who have undergone treatment for jaw malignancies may experience various side effects, such as dental issues, facial changes, or functional problems. Monitoring helps identify and manage these issues promptly.
4. **Provide Support and Guidance:** Follow-up appointments offer an opportunity for healthcare professionals to provide ongoing support, answer questions, and address any concerns the patient or their family may have.

3.6 Intraosseous Secondary (Metastatic) Malignancies

Here are key considerations for follow-up and monitoring:

1. **Frequency of Follow-Up Appointments:**
   The frequency of follow-up appointments varies depending on the patient's specific situation, the type and stage of the cancer, and the treatment received. Initially, follow-up visits are often more frequent (e.g., every few months), and they may become less frequent as time goes on.
2. **Imaging and Diagnostic Tests:**
   Imaging studies such as X-rays, CT scans, MRI scans, or PET scans may be performed during follow-up appointments to monitor the status of the jaw and surrounding structures. These tests can help detect any signs of recurrence or metastasis.
3. **Clinical Examination:**
   A thorough clinical examination by an oral and maxillofacial specialist is an essential part of each follow-up visit. This includes evaluating the oral cavity, the jaws, facial structures, and the patient's overall health.
4. **Dental and Oral Health Assessment:**
   Monitoring the patient's dental and oral health is crucial, especially if they have received radiation therapy or surgery that may affect oral structures. Regular dental check-ups are important to address any dental issues and ensure oral hygiene.
5. **Psychosocial Support:**
   Patients and their families may experience emotional and psychological challenges during the follow-up period. Supportive care and counseling services can be valuable in addressing these aspects of survivorship.
6. **Health Maintenance:**
   Encouraging patients to maintain a healthy lifestyle, including proper nutrition and regular physical activity, can contribute to their overall well-being during and after treatment.
7. **Communication:**
   Open and honest communication between the patient, their healthcare team, and their primary care physician is essential. Patients should report any new symptoms or concerns promptly.
8. **Patient Education:**
   Patients should be educated about the signs and symptoms of cancer recurrence and the importance of follow-up appointments. They should also understand the potential late effects of cancer treatment and how to manage them.
9. **Survivorship Care Plan:**
   Some healthcare institutions provide survivorship care plans, which outline the recommended follow-up schedule and provide information on managing post-treatment issues.

Follow-up and monitoring should be tailored to the individual patient's needs and circumstances. It's important for patients to actively participate in their care by attending scheduled appointments, communicating with their healthcare team, and taking steps to maintain their overall health and well-being.

(Tip 28): Regular follow-up and monitoring play a crucial role in ensuring the long-term health and quality of life for individuals who have undergone treatment for jaw malignancies.

3.6.10 Complications and Their Management

Metastatic malignancies in the jaws can lead to various complications, including severe pain, infection, and impaired oral function. A multidisciplinary team of healthcare professionals, including oral surgeons, oncologists, and palliative care specialists, is often required to manage these complications effectively.

Please refer to paragraph: Sect. 3.5.10.

3.6.11 Prognosis and Long-Term Outcomes

The prognosis for patients with jaws metastatic malignancies is generally guarded due to the advanced stage of the disease. Treatment aims to provide palliation, alleviate symptoms, and improve the patient's quality of life. Prognosis varies depending on factors such as the primary tumor type, extent of metastases, and overall health of the patient.

3.6.12 Conclusion

(Tip 29): In conclusion, metastatic malignancies affecting the jaws represent a challenging clinical scenario. Healthcare practitioners must be vigilant in considering metastatic lesions when evaluating patients with jaw abnormalities, particularly in those with a history of cancer. The management primarily revolves around palliation, pain control, and improving the patient's overall well-being.

References

1. Kochaji N. Odontogenic cysts: clinical complications and possible tumour transformation. Brussels: VUB; 2005.
2. Greer RO, Marx RE. Odontogenic and non-odontogenic cysts. Pediatric head and neck pathology. Cambridge University Press; 2016. p. 142–83.
3. Farah C, Balasubramaniam R, McCullough MJ. Contemporary oral medicine. Springer; 2019.
4. Cawson RA, Odell EW. Cawson's essentials of oral pathology and oral medicine e-book: arabic bilingual edition. Elsevier Health Sciences; 2014.

References

5. Shear M, Speight PM. Cysts of the oral and maxillofacial regions. John Wiley & Sons; 2008.
6. Regezi JA, Sciubba J, Jordan RC. Oral pathology: clinical pathologic correlations. Elsevier Health Sciences; 2016.
7. Serres ERA. Essai sur l'anatomie et la physiologie des dents, ou nouvelle théorie de la dentition. Méquignon-Marvis; 1817.
8. Neville BW, Damm DD, Allen CM, Chi AC. Oral and maxillofacial pathology. Elsevier Health Sciences; 2023.
9. Malassez L. Sur l'existence d'amas épithéliaux autour de la racine des dents chez l'homme adulte et a l'état normal:(débris épithéliaux paradentaires). G. Masson; 1885.
10. Kochaji N. Inflammatory odontogenic cyst on an osseointegrated implant: a peri-implant cyst? New entity proposed. Dent Med Probl. 2017;54(3):303–6.
11. Nanci A. Ten Cate's oral histology-e-book: development, structure, and function. Elsevier Health Sciences; 2017.
12. El-Naggar AK, Chan JKC, Grandis JR, Takata T, Slootweg PJ. WHO classification of head and neck tumours. International Agency for Research on Cancer; 2017.
13. Odell EW. Cawson's essentials of oral pathology and oral medicine e-book: Cawson's essentials of oral pathology and oral medicine e-book. Elsevier Health Sciences; 2017.
14. Kochaji N, Goossens A, Geerts A, Bottenberg P. PTCH expression in odontogenic cysts, a cause of pathogenesis or reason for clinical complication. Oral Oncol EXTRA. 2005;41(10):284–8.
15. Regezi JA, Sciubba J, Jordan RCK. Oral pathology—e-book: oral pathology—e-book. Elsevier Health Sciences; 2011.
16. Xiao X, Dai J-W, Li Z, Zhang W. Pathological fracture of the mandible caused by radicular cyst: a case report and literature review. Medicine. 2018;97(50):e13529.
17. Consolo U, Bellini P, Lizio G. Trans-nasal endoscopic marsupialization of a voluminous radicular cyst involving maxillary sinus and nasal cavity: a case report and a literature review on this surgical approach. Oral Maxillofac Surg Cases. 2018;4(3):91–6.
18. Coletti D, Ord R. Treatment rationale for pathological fractures of the mandible: a series of 44 fractures. Int J Oral Maxillofac Surg. 2008;37(3):215–22.
19. Sakkas N, Schoen R, Schulze D, Otten J-E, Schmelzeisen R. Obturator after marsupialization of a recurrence of a radicular cyst of the mandible. Oral Surg Oral Med Oral Pathol Oral Radiol Endod. 2007;103(1):e16–8.
20. Sharma P, Singh S, Mandlik J, Handa A, Khan N, Chaubey S. Management of radicular cyst by surgical enucleation: case report.
21. Carvalho FSR, Feitosa VP, da Cruz Fonseca SG, de Vasconcelos Araújo TD, Soares ECS, Fonteles CSR, et al. Physicochemical and rheological characterization of different Carnoy's solutions applied in oral and maxillofacial surgery. J Raman Spectrosc. 2017;48(10):1375–84.
22. Aguirre SE, Tyler D, Owosho AA. MAML2-rearranged primary central Mucoepidermoid carcinoma of the mandible as an incidental finding: a case report and review of the literature of molecularly confirmed cases. Case Rep Dent. 2023;2023:1.
23. Kochaji N, Goossens A, Bottenberg P. Central Mucoepidermoid carcinoma: case report, literature review for missing and available information and guideline proposal for coming case reports. Oral Oncol Extra. 2004;40(8–9):95–105.
24. Tousi F, Johannessen AC, Ljøkjel B, Løes S. Primary intraosseous carcinoma arising in a dentigerous cyst: a case report. Oral Surg. 2023;17:48.
25. Jones RS, Dillon J. Nonodontogenic cysts of the jaws and treatment in the pediatric population. Oral Maxillofac Surg Clin. 2016;28(1):31–44.
26. Rosenberger HC. Fissural cysts. Arch Otolaryngol. 1944;40(4):288–90.
27. Marx RE, Stern D. Oral and maxillofacial pathology: a rationale for diagnosis and treatment. Quintessence Publishing Company; 2012.
28. Lewandowska AM, Rudzki M, Rudzki S, Lewandowski T, Laskowska B. Environmental risk factors for cancer-review paper. Ann Agric Environ Med. 2018;26(1):1–7.
29. Chen Y, Williams V, Filippova M, Filippov V, Duerksen-Hughes P. Viral carcinogenesis: factors inducing DNA damage and virus integration. Cancers. 2014;6(4):2155–86.

30. Tamgadge S, Modak N, Tamgadge AP, Bhalerao S. Intraosseous malignant peripheral nerve sheath tumor of maxilla: a case report with review of the literature. Dent Res J. 2014;11(3):405.
31. Reddy PB, Reddy BS, Prasad N, Kumar GK, Rajnikanth M. An unusual case report of primary intraosseous carcinoma impersonating as missing mandible. Int J Oral Maxillofac Pathol. 2012;3(3):41–5.
32. Kochaji N. Maintining oral health of cancer patient in dental office. Damascus. 2007;
33. Kumar V, Abbas AK, Aster JC, Deyrup AT. Robbins & Kumar basic pathology, e-book: Robbins & Kumar basic pathology, e-book. Elsevier Health Sciences; 2022.

General Benefits

4

4.1 Can Radicular Cysts Be Healed by Endodontic Treatment?

Now coming to the point that has endless debate in the literature: can endodontic treatment heal radicular cyst?

Endodontics say yes, and argue that large periapical lesions were healed completely on radiographs, oral surgeons say no, it cannot be healed by endodontic treatment and it needs surgical intervention to remove the cystic epithelium.

Later on endodontics differ in describing two subtypes of radicular cyst, the true and bay; let us see what these two terms are:

We already know that odontogenic cysts are true cysts, meaning they have epithelium and this epithelium is of odontogenic source. If the *trigger* of proliferation for these odontogenic epithelial traces of the jaws is known to be the inflammation, then the odontogenic cyst is classified as inflammatory odontogenic cyst, and if the trigger is not known, the cyst is known as developmental odontogenic cyst [1, 2].

Radicular cyst from this point of view is a true odontogenic inflammatory cyst, and it has three subtypes depending on its topographical location to the responsible tooth:

- If it starts on the apex foremen at the far end of the pulp (the apex), then it is called *periapical cyst*.
- If it originates on a secondary canal of the necrotic pulp on the lateral wall of the tooth, then it is called **lateral cyst.**
- If the responsible tooth is completely removed and the cyst is left behind, then it is called **residual cyst**.

Based on the above criteria periapical cyst's full name should be true odontogenic inflammatory radicular periapical cyst.

© The Author(s), under exclusive license to Springer Nature Switzerland AG 2024   145
N. Kochaji, *Clinical Oral Pathology*,
https://doi.org/10.1007/978-3-031-53755-4_4

Later on, endodontics mention two subtypes of periapical cyst, the one that has a complete true lumen lined by complete epithelial circle called **true radicular cyst**, and the one that has an open in the cystic lining toward the apex foramen called **bay radicular cyst**.

They claim that the true odontogenic inflammatory radicular periapical bay cyst can be healed by endodontic treatment; the philosophical thinking is based on two theories:

1. The material used in filling root canal causes degeneration in the epithelial cells and thus results in the cyst being healed.
2. The initial cause of the cyst formation which is the necrotic pulp is removed.

Now we have to discuss these two arguments:

1. To be frank there is some periapical radiolucent lesions of considerable size that has been reported to be healed on endodontic treatment only, but it is unsure if they were radicular cyst of whatsoever subtype! It is reported that periapical lesions with well-known radiographic features have been healed, but there is no one histological examination for any of these cases; thus the first argument is still a theory without scientific proof.
2. The second argument about removing the source of inflammation neglects two major scientific points:
   (a) Cyst formation is initiated by a "trigger" and the effect of the trigger once set on cannot be revised (please see cyst formation paragraph in Chap. 3 of this book).
   (b) Residual cyst's existence, and growing, is the top proof that removing the source of inflammation cannot heal inflammatory odontogenic cysts. This cyst which was once a normal radicular cyst loses its initial trigger, still the epithelial lining keeps proliferating and expanding the cystic lesion.

However, the question still exists:

What about the documented cases of radiolucent healed lesions?

It is well known that the body defends itself against the inflammatory process in the necrotic pulp by closing the apex with a tissue composed of four components:

- Fibers and fibroblasts (to build a wall as a separator between the dead area (the necrotic pulp) and the living body (the human being).
- Foam cells (to seal completely this wall structure).
- WBC (to monitor any bypass of the wall).
- Newly formed capillaries (to have nutrition to maintain the structure).

These four components together form the basic line of defenses against pulp chronic inflammation called *periapical granuloma.*

Some times and by pure chance rests of Malassez are trapped inside this newly formed defense structure, and if the inflammatory process is not broken by good endodontic treatment, these epithelial remnants are activated to form radicular cyst.

> (Tip 1): As a conclusion, endodontic treatment can heal periapical granulomas of whatsoever size, that is, even the huge one; this explains the success cases of radiolucent lesion recovery after endodontic treatment. But radicular cyst of whatsoever subtype cannot be healed.

This leads us to the next point: how can I deal with a radiolucent lesion on the apex of a tooth?

4.2 Algorithms for Dealing with Unilocular Radiolucent Lesion

4.2.1 Algorithm for Managing Unilocular Radiolucent Lesions

1. Is the tooth vital or non-vital?
   (a) Tooth is non-vital (either endodontically treated or not): The management depends on two factors: first, the size of the lesion, and second, the quality of the endodontic treatment, which is of lesser importance.
   - Small lesion + poor endodontic treatment or non-treated tooth: The first intervention is endodontic treatment followed by periapical radiographic monitoring, preferably digital to reduce radiation dose. If the lesion is healing, then the treatment is sufficient and no further procedure is required.
   - Small lesion + good endodontic treatment: Ask the patient, "When was the treatment done?"
     - If this is a new treatment for a previously treated tooth (retreatment), monitor for changes in size.
       No change or decrease in size = Continue monitoring.
       Increase in size = Surgical intervention + histological examination.
     - If it's an old but good treatment, continue monitoring.
   - Large lesion regardless of the quality of endodontic treatment: A diagnostic aspiration biopsy is essential.
     - If fluid is present = The lesion is cystic = Surgical removal + histological analysis.
     - No fluid:
       Poor treatment = Retreatment + monitoring.
       Good treatment = Surgical removal + histological analysis.

> (Tip 2): The management of a radiolucent lesion associated with an erupted and non-vital tooth entails the combination of treatment, surgery, radiographic findings, and histological examination to best serve the patient. One should not negate the other.

> (Tip 3): The disaster is when there's a lesion unrelated to a non-vital tooth but coincidentally associated with a tooth that's either endodontically treated or non-vital.

(b) Tooth is vital: Though the probability of such a lesion is less than that of a radiolucent lesion on a non-vital tooth, we enter worse diagnostic considerations. The mildest possibility is the cementoblastoma in its initial formation, followed by developmental odontogenic cysts, odontogenic and non-odontogenic tumors, and ending with malignancies either primary or metastasis to the jaws. Each of the above had a separate section in Chap. 3.

4.3 Four Main Lesions That a Dentist May Encounter Frequently in Daily Dental Practice

4.3.1 Radicular Cyst

4.3.1.1 Introduction

A radicular cyst, also known as a periapical cyst, is a common type of odontogenic cyst that develops at the apex (tip) of a non-vital (dead) tooth [1, 2]. These cysts are usually associated with chronic dental infections and often require dental and surgical intervention for resolution. This comprehensive scientific text will provide an in-depth overview of radicular cysts, including their etiology, clinical presentation, diagnosis, histopathology, treatment, and potential complications (Fig. 4.1: case of radicular cyst).

4.3.1.2 Etiology

Radicular cysts primarily originate from inflammatory processes within the pulp of a tooth and its periapical tissues. Several factors contribute to their development:

1. **Chronic Infection:** The most common cause is a long-standing dental infection, which may result from untreated dental caries, trauma, or periodontal disease.
2. **Necrotic Pulp:** The death of pulp tissue within the tooth triggers an inflammatory response, leading to cyst formation.

4.3 Four Main Lesions That a Dentist May Encounter Frequently in Daily Dental...   149

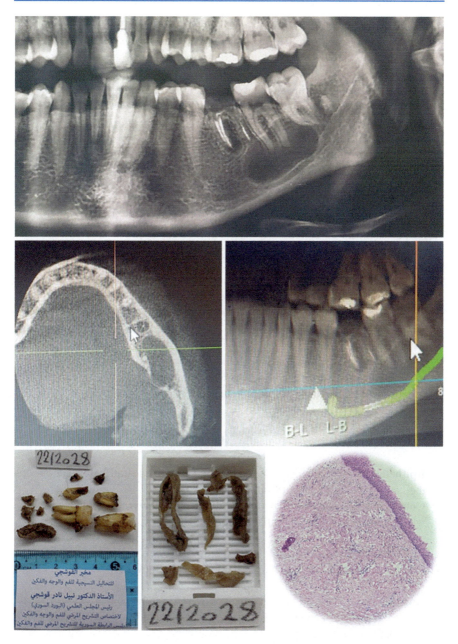

Fig. 4.1 Radicular cyst case. On radiograph, look how it preserved cortical bone, and the mandibular alveolar nerve

4.3.1.3 Clinical Presentation

Radicular cysts can manifest with various clinical features:

1. **Asymptomatic:** In many cases, these cysts are asymptomatic and are discovered incidentally during routine dental examinations or radiographic evaluations.
2. **Pain and Swelling:** If the cyst becomes infected or enlarges significantly, it can cause localized pain and swelling in the affected area.
3. **Sinus Tract:** Sometimes, a chronic sinus tract (gum boil) may form near the affected tooth, allowing pus drainage.
4. **Tooth Discoloration:** Discoloration of the tooth may occur if the cyst affects the development of permanent teeth [2–4].

4.3.1.4 Diagnosis

Accurate diagnosis of radicular cysts involves a combination of clinical, radiographic, and histopathological assessments [2, 3, 5]:

1. **Clinical Examination:** A thorough clinical examination, including the evaluation of symptoms and physical findings, is essential.
2. **Radiographic Evaluation:** Dental radiographs, such as periapical or panoramic radiographs, are crucial for visualizing the cyst's location, size, and relationship with the affected tooth.
3. **Histopathological Examination:** A biopsy or surgical excision of the cyst lining is often necessary for definitive diagnosis. Histopathological examination reveals the cystic lining and its epithelial components.

4.3.1.5 Histopathology

Histologically, radicular cysts typically exhibit the following features [2, 6]:

1. **Epithelial Lining:** The cyst is lined by non-keratinized stratified squamous epithelium, often with a layer of inflammatory cells.
2. **Connective Tissue Wall:** The cyst wall consists of fibrous connective tissue, which may contain chronic inflammatory cells.

4.3.1.6 Treatment

The primary treatment for radicular cysts is surgical removal [4, 7]:

1. **Apicoectomy:** This procedure involves removing the apical portion of the affected tooth's root and the associated cystic tissue. In some cases, extraction of the tooth may be necessary.
2. **Endodontic Therapy:** After cyst removal or apicoectomy, root canal therapy may be performed on the affected tooth to prevent future infections.
3. **Histopathological Examination:** The excised tissue should be sent for histopathological examination to confirm the diagnosis and rule out any malignant changes.

4.3.1.7 Complications

Untreated or inadequately managed radicular cysts can lead to several complications:

1. **Infection:** Persistent infection can cause pain, swelling, and potential systemic issues.
2. **Tooth Loss:** In severe cases, untreated radicular cysts may lead to tooth loss.

4.3.1.8 Prognosis

The prognosis for patients with radicular cysts is generally favorable when promptly diagnosed and appropriately treated. Surgical removal of the cyst, often in conjunction with endodontic therapy, effectively resolves the issue, and recurrence is rare [4, 7].

> (Tip 4): Conclusion: Radicular cysts are common odontogenic cysts that typically develop at the apex of non-vital teeth in response to chronic dental infections. Early diagnosis through clinical examination and radiography is essential for successful treatment and to prevent potential complications. Surgical removal and appropriate dental interventions are the primary treatment modalities, leading to a favorable prognosis for affected individuals.

4.3.2 Dentigerous Cyst

A dentigerous cyst, also known as a follicular cyst, is a common type of odontogenic cyst that forms around the crown of an unerupted tooth. These cysts are typically benign and usually associated with impacted, unerupted, or partially erupted teeth. This comprehensive scientific text will provide an in-depth overview of dentigerous cysts, including their etiology, clinical presentation, diagnosis, histopathology, treatment, and potential complications (Figs. 4.2 and 4.3: cases of dentigerous cyst).

4.3.2.1 Introduction

Dentigerous cysts are a type of odontogenic cyst, which means they originate from tooth-forming tissues. They are often found incidentally during routine dental examinations or when investigating the cause of dental impactions. Understanding the various aspects of dentigerous cysts is crucial for dental practitioners, oral surgeons, and pathologists [2, 3, 8].

4.3.2.2 Etiology

The exact cause of dentigerous cysts remains unclear, but several factors contribute to their development [4, 8]:

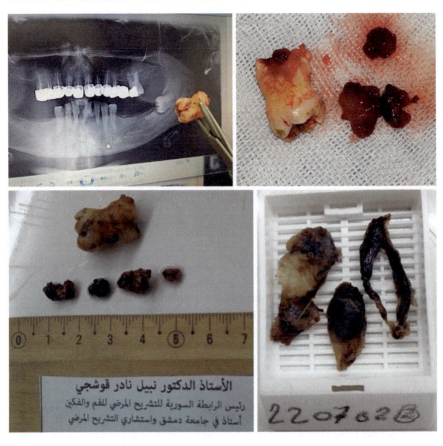

Fig. 4.2 Dentigerous cyst case. Old theory that distinguishes between dentigerous cyst and dilated dental follicle depending on radiographs can be proven wrong with this case of dentigerous cyst

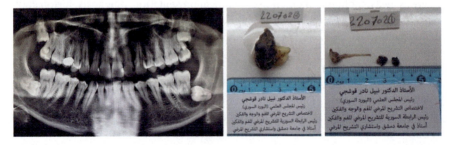

Fig. 4.3 Dentigerous cyst case. The patient came with the chief complaint of acute pulpal pain from the second molar; it's obvious that the impacted third molar and its dentigerous cyst are the cause

1. **Developmental Factors:** Dentigerous cysts frequently arise due to a developmental abnormality during tooth formation, where the cyst forms around the crown of an unerupted tooth. The most commonly affected teeth are third molars (wisdom teeth) and canines.
2. **Genetic Predisposition:** There may be a genetic predisposition for some individuals to develop dentigerous cysts.

4.3.2.3 Clinical Presentation

Dentigerous cysts may be asymptomatic and discovered incidentally on radiographs. However, they can lead to various clinical manifestations [2, 3, 9]:

1. **Swelling:** A painless, slow-growing swelling may be noticeable in the affected area.
2. **Displacement of Adjacent Teeth:** The cyst's growth can cause displacement or resorption of adjacent teeth, leading to malocclusion.
3. **Pain and Discomfort:** In some cases, pain and discomfort may occur if the cyst becomes infected or enlarges significantly.
4. **Facial Deformity:** In severe cases, untreated cysts can cause facial deformity.

4.3.2.4 Diagnosis

Accurate diagnosis of dentigerous cysts involves a combination of clinical, radiographic, and histopathological assessment [10]:

1. **Clinical Examination:** A thorough clinical examination, including palpation and inspection of the affected area, is crucial to assess the size and characteristics of the swelling.
2. **Radiographic Evaluation:** Dental radiographs, such as panoramic radiographs or cone-beam computed tomography (CBCT), are essential for visualizing the cyst's size, location, and its relationship with the involved tooth.
3. **Histopathological Examination:** To confirm the diagnosis, a biopsy or surgical excision of the cyst lining is necessary. Histopathological examination reveals the cystic lining and its epithelial components.

4.3.2.5 Histopathology

Histologically, dentigerous cysts typically exhibit the following features [3, 4]:

1. **Epithelial Lining:** The cyst is lined by non-keratinized stratified squamous epithelium, often with a thin layer of cuboidal or columnar cells.
2. **Connective Tissue Wall:** The cyst wall consists of fibrous connective tissue.

4.3.2.6 Treatment

The primary treatment for dentigerous cysts is surgical removal [2, 4, 6]:

1. **Enucleation:** This procedure involves the complete removal of the cyst along with the unerupted tooth, if necessary.
2. **Marsupialization:** In cases where the cyst is large or associated with important structures, marsupialization may be performed to decompress the cyst and allow for gradual reduction in size before complete removal.
3. **Histopathological Examination:** The excised tissue should be sent for histopathological examination to confirm the diagnosis and rule out any malignant changes.

4.3.2.7 Complications

While dentigerous cysts are usually benign, they can lead to complications if left untreated [9, 11]:

1. **Infection:** Cyst infection can cause pain, swelling, and systemic symptoms.
2. **Bone Resorption:** Prolonged cyst growth can lead to resorption of adjacent bone, potentially causing facial deformities.
3. **Pathologic Fractures:** Severe cysts may weaken the jawbone, increasing the risk of pathologic fractures.
4. **Neoplastic Transformation:** Dentigerous cysts neoplastic transfomation into unocystic ameloblastoma is documented in the literature.
5. **Malignant Transformation:** Malignant transformation into mucoepidermoid carcinoma and sqoaumous cell carcinoma is also reported.

4.3.2.8 Prognosis

The prognosis for patients with dentigerous cysts is generally excellent when promptly diagnosed and treated. Complete surgical removal typically resolves the issue, and recurrence is rare [3, 9].

> (Tip 5): Conclusion: Dentigerous cysts are common odontogenic cysts that typically form around unerupted teeth. Early diagnosis through clinical examination and radiography is crucial for successful treatment and to prevent potential complications. Surgical removal, often accompanied by histopathological examination, is the primary treatment modality, and it generally leads to a favorable prognosis for affected individuals.

4.3.3 Odontogenic Keratocyst

4.3.3.1 Introduction

Odontogenic keratocysts (OKCs) are a type of developmental odontogenic cysts that originate from the remnants of dental lamina or basal cells of the oral

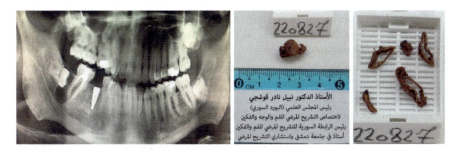

Fig. 4.4 Odontogenic keratocyst case. On radiograph, macroscopically and upon sectioning it looks like dentigerous cyst, still the microscope lens has another point of view with this odontogenic keratocyst

epithelium. They are characterized by their unique histological features and clinical behavior. This comprehensive scientific text will provide an in-depth overview of odontogenic keratocysts, including their etiology, clinical presentation, diagnosis, histopathology, treatment, and potential complications (Fig. 4.4: OKC case).

4.3.3.2 Etiology
The exact cause of odontogenic keratocysts is not fully understood, but they are believed to arise due to developmental abnormalities and genetic factors [3, 4]:

1. **Developmental Factors:** OKCs develop from dental lamina remnants, which are involved in tooth formation. They can occur sporadically or as part of inherited syndromes such as Gorlin-Goltz syndrome.
2. **Genetic Predisposition:** Some individuals may have a genetic predisposition to develop OKCs, particularly in cases of Gorlin-Goltz syndrome.

4.3.3.3 Clinical Presentation
Odontogenic keratocysts can present with various clinical features [2, 3]:

1. **Asymptomatic:** OKCs are often asymptomatic and may be discovered incidentally during routine dental radiographic examinations.
2. **Painless Swelling:** Larger cysts can cause painless swelling in the affected area, which may be noticeable on the face or inside the mouth.
3. **Tooth Displacement:** OKCs can displace adjacent teeth, leading to malocclusion.
4. **Bone Expansion:** As they grow, these cysts can cause expansion and thinning of the jawbone.

4.3.3.4 Diagnosis
Accurate diagnosis of odontogenic keratocysts involves a combination of clinical, radiographic, and histopathological assessments [2, 4, 12]:

1. **Clinical Examination:** A thorough clinical examination, including inspection and palpation of the affected area, is important for assessing the size and characteristics of the swelling.
2. **Radiographic Evaluation:** Dental radiographs, such as panoramic radiographs or cone-beam computed tomography (CBCT), are essential for visualizing the cyst's location, size, and any associated changes in bone structure.
3. **Histopathological Examination:** A biopsy or surgical excision of the cyst lining is necessary for definitive diagnosis. Histopathological examination reveals the characteristic features of OKCs, including a stratified squamous epithelial lining with a distinct keratin layer.

4.3.3.5 Histopathology

Histologically, odontogenic keratocysts are characterized by several unique features [3, 4]:

1. **Thin Epithelial Lining:** The cyst is lined by a thin, uniform layer of stratified squamous epithelium.
2. **Keratinization:** OKCs typically exhibit prominent keratinization, with a distinctive corrugated or "parakeratin" layer on the luminal surface.
3. **Palisaded Basal Cells:** The basal cell layer of the epithelium is often palisaded, contributing to the characteristic appearance.
4. **Epithelial Lining Separation:** The epithelium of this cyst might be separated from the underlined connective tissue causing increasing recurrence rates.
5. **Daughter Cyst:** Daughter cysts can be seen in the cystic wall.

4.3.3.6 Treatment

The treatment of odontogenic keratocysts generally involves surgical intervention [2, 4, 13]:

1. **Enucleation:** Surgical removal of the cyst and its lining is the primary treatment. It's essential to remove the entire cyst to prevent recurrence.
2. **Carnoy's Solution:** In some cases, after enucleation, the surgical site may be treated with Carnoy's solution to decrease the risk of recurrence.
3. **Regular Follow-up:** Patients should undergo regular follow-up examinations and radiographic assessments to monitor for recurrence, as OKCs have a higher tendency to recur compared to other odontogenic cysts.

4.3.3.7 Complications

Complications associated with odontogenic keratocysts may include the following [4, 14]:

1. **Recurrence:** OKCs have a relatively high recurrence rate, making long-term follow-up essential.
2. **Pathologic Fracture:** In cases of extensive bone expansion, pathologic fractures may occur.
3. **Neoplastic Transformation:** As a developmental odontogenic cysts, OKC cases of neoplastic transformation has been reported in the literature.

4.3 Four Main Lesions That a Dentist May Encounter Frequently in Daily Dental... 157

4.3.3.8 Prognosis
The prognosis for patients with odontogenic keratocysts is generally favorable with appropriate surgical treatment and follow-up. However, due to their higher recurrence rate compared to other cysts, ongoing monitoring is crucial [2, 14].

> (Tip 6): Conclusion: Odontogenic keratocysts are distinctive odontogenic cysts that arise from developmental remnants of dental lamina or basal cells. Timely diagnosis through clinical examination and radiography is essential for successful treatment and long-term follow-up to monitor for recurrence. Surgical removal, often accompanied by the use of Carnoy's solution, is the primary treatment modality, and it provides a favorable prognosis for affected individuals.

4.3.4 Ameloblastoma

4.3.4.1 Introduction
Ameloblastomas are benign but locally aggressive tumors that originate from odontogenic epithelium, particularly from the cells that form tooth enamel (ameloblasts). They are among the most common odontogenic tumors and can cause significant oral and maxillofacial complications [15]. This comprehensive scientific text will provide an in-depth overview of ameloblastomas, including their etiology, clinical presentation, diagnosis, histopathology, treatment, and potential complications (Fig. 4.5: Ameloblastoma case).

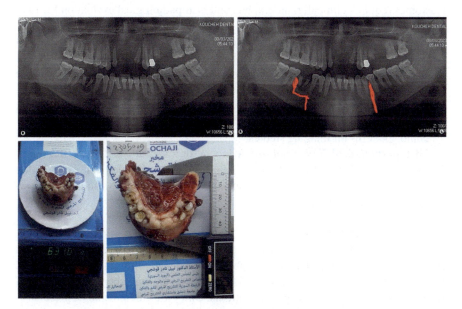

Fig. 4.5 Ameloblastoma case. The red lines were drawn by the oral maxillofacial surgeon who performed the resection of this case of recurrent ameloblastoma

4.3.4.2 Etiology

The exact cause of ameloblastomas is not fully understood, but several factors may contribute to their development [4]:

- **Developmental Factors:** Ameloblastomas are thought to arise from remnants of odontogenic epithelium or from the enamel organ during tooth development.
- **Genetic Factors:** Genetic mutations and alterations may play a role in the development of ameloblastomas, but specific genetic markers are still under investigation.

4.3.4.3 Clinical Presentation

Ameloblastomas can present with a variety of clinical features [2, 16]:

1. **Asymptomatic:** Many ameloblastomas are asymptomatic and are discovered incidentally during routine dental radiographic examinations.
2. **Painless Swelling:** Larger tumors can cause painless swelling in the jaw or oral cavity, which may lead to facial deformity.
3. **Displacement of Teeth:** Ameloblastomas can displace or resorb adjacent teeth, leading to malocclusion.
4. **Paresthesia:** Tumors involving the inferior alveolar nerve may cause paresthesia (numbness or tingling) in the lower lip or chin.

4.3.4.4 Diagnosis

Ameloblastomas exhibit a diverse range of clinical and radiographic presentations, making their diagnosis and management challenging. Accurate diagnosis of ameloblastomas requires clinical, radiographic, and histopathological evaluation [2, 17]:

1. **Clinical Examination:** Thorough clinical examination, including palpation and assessment of the extent of the swelling and facial deformity, is crucial.
2. **Radiographic Evaluation:** Dental radiographs, CT scans, or MRI scans are essential for visualizing the tumor's location, size, and its relationship with surrounding structures. Radiographically, ameloblastomas appear as well-defined, multilocular radiolucent lesions with characteristic "soap bubble" or "honeycomb" patterns on imaging studies.
3. **Histopathological Examination:** A biopsy or surgical excision of the tumor tissue is necessary for definitive diagnosis. Histopathological examination reveals the characteristic features of ameloblastomas, such as islands and strands of odontogenic epithelium.

4.3.4.5 Histopathology

Histologically, ameloblastomas exhibit different subtypes, including conventional (solid/multicystic), unicystic, and peripheral types, each with distinct microscopic features. Conventional ameloblastoma is the most common subtype and is characterized by solid or multicystic growth patterns. Unicystic ameloblastoma presents as a unilocular cystic lesion with an intraluminal or mural proliferation of ameloblastoma-like epithelium. Peripheral ameloblastoma involves the soft tissues surrounding the tooth-bearing areas and is often associated with the gingiva [4, 15, 16, 18].

All amoleblastomas types consist of islands or strands of odontogenic epithelium *resembling* ameloblasts.

4.3.4.6 Treatment

Ameloblastomas are notorious for their locally aggressive behavior and high recurrence rates. Treatment options may include enucleation and curettage for less aggressive lesions, segmental resection for more extensive cases. Long-term follow-up is critical due to their potential for recurrence [2, 4, 18, 19].

The treatment of ameloblastomas typically involves aggressive surgical intervention:

1. **En Bloc Resection:** The preferred treatment is complete surgical removal of the tumor, including a margin of healthy tissue to minimize the risk of recurrence.
2. **Reconstruction:** Following tumor resection, reconstruction of the affected area may be necessary, which can involve bone grafts, plates, or other techniques to restore facial symmetry and function.
3. **Long-Term Follow-up:** Due to the potential for recurrence, long-term follow-up with clinical examinations and imaging is essential.

4.3.4.7 Complications

Complications associated with ameloblastomas may include [4, 15]:

1. **Recurrence:** Ameloblastomas have a relatively high recurrence rate if not adequately treated.
2. **Facial Deformity:** Extensive tumors can lead to facial deformity and functional impairment.

4.3.4.8 Prognosis

The prognosis for patients with ameloblastomas is generally favorable with appropriate surgical treatment and long-term follow-up. Early diagnosis and complete surgical resection are crucial to minimize the risk of recurrence and complications [16].

4.3.4.9 Conclusion

Ameloblastomas are locally aggressive odontogenic tumors that arise from remnants of odontogenic epithelium. Timely diagnosis through clinical examination, radiography, and histopathological assessment is essential for successful treatment and long-term follow-up to monitor for recurrence. Aggressive surgical resection, often followed by reconstruction, provides a favorable prognosis for affected individuals.

4.4 Are Rare Lesions Really Rare?

During a quarter of a century in my career as an oral maxillofacial pathologist, I encountered really rare lesions, documented them all, and published a few:

1. Rare case of central capillary hemangioma.

   Here every clinical, radiographical sign was pushing toward the diagnosis of radicular cyst, still because the bleeding during surgical intervention to remove the innocent radicular cyst prompted the general dentist to ask for histological examination [20].
2. Rare case of glandular odontogenic cyst.

   Here the initial diagnosis was developmental cyst, but because of the nervous signs that should not exist, a histological study was performed. Again, if everything was non-suspicious nobody would know about this case, and it was going to be recorded as cystic lesion [21]!
3. Case No. 33 for central lipoma of the jaws.

   Here it was barely seen as radiolucent lesion on a partially erupted third molar; even the surgeon who performed the operation thought it is only a thickness in the follicle surrounding the tooth [22]!
4. Case No. 11 for intraosseous bilateral ossifying fibroma.

   Because of the symmetric appearance, doubts were raised here. It is not common that a tumor develops on both sides of the jaws, with an exception to cherubism; still the clinical and radiographical signs were very far from central giant cell appearance, without histopathological study, and if it was not documented, no human would know about this case [23]!
5. Case no. 4 of odontogenic keratocyst in masticator muscle.

   When the head and neck surgeon consulted me about this case, and before the routine pathological process was completed I was thinking about parasite cystic lesion, although it's rare, but under the lens of the microscope an extremely rare case was detected—OKC in the cheek muscles [24]!
6. First case was of ameloblastoma causing double vision that was cured by surgical removal of the tumor.

   The patient's only complaint was an increasing double vision. That was the only sign to ask for a radiograph, and it showed a lesion in the maxilla. When an excisional biopsy was performed and it turned out to be ameloblastoma, the double vision was cured and the patient refused to do further surgery as his vison was restored [25]!

The case that I will never publish as a case report goes as follows:

A patient came complaining of pain in first mandibular molar area, and an endodontic treatment was performed. Panoramic radiograph showed a uniocular radiolucent lesion. This lesion was diagnosed radiographically only as radicular cyst, and just as thousands of similar cases all over the world were treated, the teeth was extracted and the lesion was surgically removed without histopathological examination.

Later an implant was inserted in the extracted tooth socket, but at follow-up it turned out to be a failing implant; this time the implant was removed and the lesion

4.4 Are Rare Lesions Really Rare?

was submitted for histopathological evaluation, and it turned to be ossifying fibroma!

Please look carefully at the following figures (Fig. 4.6). Three seirial radiographs, the mandibular left first molar with a radioluceny at the apex was endodontic treated, extracted, and later an implant was inserted. After implant failure an excisonal biopsy was performed, and the radiolucent lesion was diagoned as ossyfing fibroma!

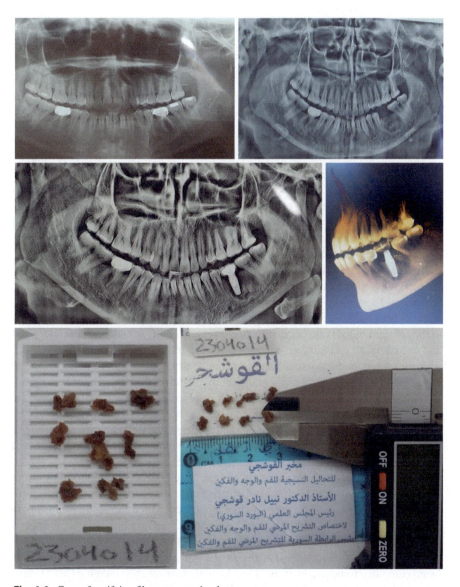

Fig. 4.6 Case of ossifying fibroma on an implant

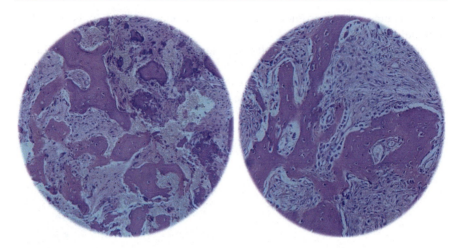

Fig. 4.6 (continued)

This case is one of the reasons why we wrote the first paragraph of this part of the guideline was written to explain such cases shown in figure 4.6.

For discussing such cases the idea of this book came through my mind. Dentists have to know the importance of clinical oral pathology in their daily dental practice, and for such cases the emphasis all over the book was about algorithm of logical thinking and that the intraosseous lesions of the jaws are not only either radicular cyst or dentigerous cyst.

To clarify the idea, the human jaws, composed of the mandible and the maxilla, are integral components of the oral and facial anatomy. While they primarily serve the crucial functions of mastication and speech, they can also be susceptible to a wide array of pathologies and lesions. One commonly held belief is that rare lesions in the jaws are indeed rare occurrences. However, delving into the intricacies of oral and maxillofacial medicine reveals that this assumption may not hold true.

Rare lesions in the jaws, although uncommon in comparison to more prevalent oral conditions, do exist and can manifest in a variety of forms. These lesions can encompass a spectrum of etiologies, including developmental anomalies, neoplastic growths, cystic formations, and inflammatory processes. While they may not be encountered as frequently as common dental issues like dental caries (cavities) or gingival disease; their diagnosis and management remain crucial within the realm of oral healthcare.

One reason why these lesions may appear "rare" is because they often present with non-specific clinical symptoms. Patients may initially experience mild discomfort, swelling, or an unusual sensation in the jaw area, which can easily be attributed to more common dental ailments. As a result, these rare lesions might go unnoticed or misdiagnosed until they progress to a more advanced stage.

Furthermore, advancements in diagnostic imaging techniques, such as cone-beam computed tomography (CBCT) and magnetic resonance imaging (MRI), have improved our ability to detect and differentiate rare lesions in the jaws. These technologies provide clinicians with a more detailed view of the affected area, aiding in the accurate diagnosis and treatment planning for these conditions.

On top of reasons of their rarity is that many if not a lot of oral cases are diagnosed relying on clinical examination only, or clinical and radiographical examinations. Many rare cases associated with impacted teeth are being diagnosed as dentigerous cysts, surgically removed, and thrown away; the area got healed, but nobody knows what really the diagnosis was!

> (Tip 7): Day after day, I become more convinced that the rarity of cases is solely due to neglecting the histological examination and documentation of the lesions.

In conclusion, while rare lesions in the jaws may not be as prevalent as more common dental conditions, they do exist and should not be underestimated. Dentists and oral and maxillofacial surgeons must maintain a high level of clinical suspicion and employ advanced diagnostic tools to identify and manage these rare lesions effectively. Early detection and appropriate treatment are essential to ensure the best possible outcomes for patients facing these uncommon challenges in oral healthcare.

For example, look at this case that I have never published:

4.5 Short Stories

4.5.1 The Painful Sorrow

Dr. Sarah Mitchell was renowned in the field of clinical oral pathology. Her passion for unraveling the mysteries hidden within patients' mouths had led her to the forefront of her profession. Despite her expertise, there was one case that had eluded her for years—a perplexing oral disease that refused to reveal its secrets.

The case belonged to Mr. Robert Jennings, a retired schoolteacher with a penchant for gardening. Robert had visited countless doctors and dentists over the years, seeking an answer to the persistent pain in his mouth. He described it as a gnawing sensation, a burning discomfort that had slowly but steadily worsened.

Dr. Mitchell had pored over Robert's medical history and dental records, conducted numerous examinations, and even sought second opinions from colleagues. Yet, the source of Robert's agony remained elusive. It wasn't an infection, a tumor, or any known disease. The tests were inconclusive, and the treatments ineffective.

Late one evening, after another long day at the lab, Dr. Mitchell sat in her office, surrounded by stacks of research papers and textbooks. Frustration weighed on her shoulders. She was on the brink of giving up, feeling like she had reached the limits of her knowledge.

Then, an idea struck her like a bolt of lightning. She decided to take a different approach. Instead of focusing solely on the physical aspects of Robert's condition, she began to explore the emotional and psychological factors that might contribute to his pain.

She asked Robert about his life, his experiences, and any stressors he had encountered. It was during this conversation that Robert shared a deeply personal story. He had lost his wife to cancer a few years ago, a devastating blow that had left him emotionally shattered.

As Dr. Mitchell listened, she realized that Robert's pain might be a manifestation of his grief—a condition rarely considered in clinical oral pathology. She referred him to a therapist to address his emotional turmoil while continuing to monitor his oral health.

Over time, as Robert's emotional healing progressed, his oral pain began to subside. Dr. Mitchell's innovative approach had led to a diagnosis that had eluded her for years—psychosomatic oral pain.

The case of Mr. Robert Jennings became a turning point in the field of clinical oral pathology. Dr. Mitchell's experience highlighted the importance of considering the holistic well-being of patients, not just their physical symptoms. It was a reminder that sometimes, the answers lie not only within the tissues of the mouth but within the depths of the human heart.

4.5.2 The Mysterious Lesion

Dr. Amelia Williams was a brilliant oral maxillofacial surgeon with a reputation for solving the most perplexing cases. She had seen a myriad of oral conditions throughout her career, but one case in particular had left her scratching her head.

It was a damp, gloomy morning when Mrs. Eleanor Turner walked into Dr. Williams' clinic. Eleanor was a middle-aged woman who exuded grace and composure despite her obvious discomfort. She explained to Dr. Williams that she had been experiencing a persistent lesion on her tongue for several months. It was a small, white patch that seemed innocuous at first glance, but it had grown increasingly painful.

Dr. Williams examined the lesion carefully, taking biopsy samples for analysis. She sent the samples to oral maxillofacial pathology laboratory and awaited the results with bated breath. Days turned into weeks, and the tests came back inconclusive. The lesion displayed abnormal cell growth, but it didn't match any known oral pathology.

Undeterred, Dr. Williams delved into Eleanor's medical history. She asked about her lifestyle, diet, and any recent changes that might offer clues. Eleanor mentioned that she had recently started a new job at a winery and had been sampling various wines as part of her role.

A thought crossed Dr. Williams' mind. Could the lesion be related to something in the wines Eleanor had been tasting? She decided to conduct an experiment. She obtained samples of the wines Eleanor had been exposed to and enlisted the help of a colleague, a sommelier with an acute palate.

4.5 Short Stories

Together, they meticulously analyzed the wines, scrutinizing every element. To their astonishment, they discovered that one of the wines contained a rare and highly reactive compound that had been overlooked in the initial assessments. This compound had the potential to cause cellular changes when in contact with oral tissues.

With this breakthrough, Dr. Williams could finally provide Eleanor with a diagnosis—chemical-induced oral hyperplasia. The lesion was a direct result of her exposure to this specific compound in the wine.

Eleanor made the necessary adjustments to her job, avoiding wines that contained the troublesome compound. As she did, her tongue gradually healed, and the pain dissipated. Dr. Williams' dedication to solving the enigmatic lesion not only relieved Eleanor's suffering but also expanded the knowledge base in clinical oral pathology.

This case served as a reminder that sometimes the answers to medical mysteries lie in unexpected places. It showcased the importance of thorough investigation, open-mindedness, and collaboration in the ever-evolving field of clinical oral pathology.

4.5.3 The Hidden Threat

Dr. Emanuel Turner was a highly respected clinical oral pathologist, renowned for her dedication to uncovering even the most concealed oral diseases. However, one particularly challenging case would test her expertise to its limits—a case where the threat lay hidden within the jaws themselves.

One spring morning, Mark Anderson walked into Dr. Turner's clinic, a man in his early forties who had recently started experiencing excruciating pain deep inside his jaw. The pain was constant, throbbing, and had begun to affect Mark's ability to eat, sleep, and even speak. Desperate for relief, he had already seen several dentists and physicians, but none could identify the source of his agony.

Dr. Turner, known for her thoroughness, started by reviewing Mark's medical history and conducting a series of examinations. Mark's jaw appeared normal on the surface, and initial X-rays showed nothing unusual. Despite the lack of evidence, Dr. Turner couldn't dismiss Mark's suffering and committed herself to getting to the bottom of the mystery.

He ordered more advanced imaging tests, including a cone beam CT scan that would provide a detailed, three-dimensional view of the jaw. It was during this scan that the hidden threat finally revealed itself—a small, nearly imperceptible mass nestled within Mark's jawbone.

The mass was nestled near a cluster of nerves, which explained the excruciating pain Mark had been enduring. Dr. Turner suspected it might be a rare and slow-growing odontogenic tumor, a type of oral tumor that originates from the tooth-forming tissues. Further biopsies and genetic testing confirmed her suspicions.

Mark underwent surgery to remove the tumor, which was caught just in time to prevent further damage. The procedure was successful, and over time, his pain subsided, and he gradually regained the ability to lead a normal life.

Dr. Turner's relentless pursuit of the elusive diagnosis had saved Mark from a potentially debilitating and life-altering condition. Her dedication to her patient's well-being, even when faced with an uncommon and hidden threat, underscored the critical importance of specialized expertise in clinical oral pathology.

Mark's story became a testament to the necessity of perseverance and advanced diagnostic techniques in the field, reminding both healthcare professionals and patients that even the most elusive conditions could be unraveled with the right expertise and determination.

4.6 Catastrophic True Case

This is a true sad story:

A male, 72 years old, consulted his dentist for a dull pain in the right upper molar area; the dentist prescribed an antibiotic and analgesic for a week, and extracted one of the molars in the area (without asking or making a radiograph of the area). Two weeks later the pain was continuous and the wound of extraction was not healed, so another course of medication was prescribed for a week.

Two months later the case was referred to an oral surgeon for advice. The case would be described as huge mass of several cementers, on radiographs it was extending to the eye!

An incisional biopsy was performed and the case was squamous cell carcinoma (Fig. 4.7).

The oral mucosal lesions will be the main topic of the second volume of this book.

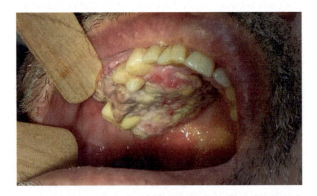

Fig. 4.7 Case of squamous cell carcinoma

References

1. Soluk-Tekkesin M, Wright JM. The World Health Organization classification of odontogenic lesions: a summary of the changes of the 2022 (5th) edition. Turk Patoloji Derg. 2022;38(2):168–84.
2. Cawson CR. In: Odell W, editor. Fundamentos de medicina y patología oral. Barcelona: Elsevier; 2017.
3. Greer RO, Marx RE. Odontogenic and non-odontogenic cysts. In: Pediatric head and neck pathology. Cambridge University Press; 2016. p. 142–83.
4. Regezi JA, Sciubba J, Jordan RC. Oral pathology: clinical pathologic correlations. Elsevier Health Sciences; 2016.
5. Ver Berne J, Saadi SB, Politis C, Jacobs R. A deep learning approach for radiological detection and classification of radicular cysts and periapical granulomas. J Dent. 2023;104581:104581.
6. Neville BW, Damm DD, Allen CM, Chi AC. Oral and maxillofacial pathology. Elsevier Health Sciences; 2015.
7. Pulatova SK, Yusupov SAJT, Science A. Enhancement treatments of methods of radicular cysts of jaw. Theor Appl Sci. 2020;5:337–40.
8. Ghafouri-Fard S, Atarbashi-Moghadam S, Taheri M. Genetic factors in the pathogenesis of ameloblastoma, dentigerous cyst and odontogenic keratocyst. Gene. 2021;771:145369.
9. Shear M, Speight PM. Cysts of the oral and maxillofacial regions. John Wiley & Sons; 2008.
10. Mei H-X, Cheng J-H, Li Y-Z, Ma H-S, Zhang K-W, Shou Y-K, et al. Advances in the application of machine learning in maxillofacial cysts and tumors. West China J Stomatol. 2020;38(6):687–91.
11. Terauchi M, Akiya S, Kumagai J, Ohyama Y, Yamaguchi SJ. An analysis of dentigerous cysts developed around a mandibular third molar by panoramic radiographs. Dent J. 2019;7(1):13.
12. Boffano P, Cavarra F, Agnone AM, Brucoli M, Ruslin M, Forouzanfar T, et al. The epidemiology and management of odontogenic keratocysts (OKCs): a European multicenter study. J Craniomaxillofac Surg. 2022;50(1):1–6.
13. Mohanty S, Dabas J, Verma A, Gupta S, Urs A, Hemavathy S, et al. Surgical management of the odontogenic keratocyst: a 20-year experience. Int J Oral Maxillofac Surg. 2021;50(9):1168–76.
14. Fidele N-B, Yueyu Z, Zhao Y, Tianfu W, Liu J, Sun Y, et al. Recurrence of odontogenic keratocysts and possible prognostic factors: review of 455 patients. Med Oral Patol Oral Cir Bucal. 2019;24(4):e491.
15. Kondamari SK, Taneeru S, Guttikonda VR, Masabattula GK. Ameloblastoma arising in the wall of dentigerous cyst: report of a rare entity. J Oral Maxillofac Pathol. 2018;22(Suppl 1):S7.
16. Evangelou Z, Zarachi A, Dumollard JM, Michel PH, Komnos I, Kastanioudakis I, et al. Maxillary ameloblastoma: a review with clinical, histological and prognostic data of a rare tumor. in vivo. 2020;34(5):2249–58.
17. Kitisubkanchana J, Reduwan NH, Poomsawat S, Pornprasertsuk-Damrongsri S, Wongchuensoontorn CJ. Odontogenic keratocyst and ameloblastoma: radiographic evaluation. Oral Radiol. 2021;37:55–65.
18. Shi HA, Ng CWB, Kwa CT, Sim QX. Ameloblastoma: a succinct review of the classification, genetic understanding and novel molecular targeted therapies. The Surg. 2021;19(4):238–43.
19. Qiao X, Shi J, Liu J, Liu J, Guo Y, Zhong MJ. Recurrence rates of intraosseous ameloblastoma cases with conservative or aggressive treatment: a systematic review and meta-analysis. Front Oncol. 2021;11:647200.

20. Kochaji N, Ajalyakeen H, Fakir A, AAS A-M. Intraosseous hemangioma of the mandible: a rare case report. Int J Surg Case Rep. 2023;109:108496.
21. Kochaji N, Alhessani S, Ibrahim S, Al-Awad AJ. Posterior mandibular glandular cyst: a rare case report. Int J Surg Case Rep. 2023;106:108169.
22. Kochaji N, Alhessani S, AHJ D. Intraosseous lipoma of the jaws: review of the literature and rare case report. Int J Surg Case Rep. 2022;101:107786.
23. Kochaji N, Darwich K, Ahmad M, Mahfuri AJ. Bilateral ossifying fibroma affecting the jaws: literature review, rare case report. Int J Surg Case Rep. 2023;106:108283.
24. Kochaji N, Alshami G, Haddad BJ. Primary odontogenic keratocyst in the cheek muscles: report of the 4th case in the world and review of peripheral OKC literature. Int J Surg Case Rep. 2023;106:108161.
25. Kochaji N, Barbar R, Al-Assaf M, Barakat CJ. Extremely rare maxillary unicystic ameloblastoma causing double vision: first case report in the middle east. Int J Surg Case Rep. 2023;109:108485.

Index

A
Adenomatoid odontogenic tumor, 55, 90
Alcohol, 10, 16, 17, 19, 30, 49, 123
Ameloblastic carcinoma, 41, 112, 123, 126, 127
Ameloblastic fibroma, 63, 72, 73
Ameloblastoma, 34, 40–41, 53, 55, 63, 70, 72–75, 93, 112, 157–159

B
Brush biopsy, 11
Buccal bifurcation cyst, 57

C
Calcifying epithelial odontogenic tumor, *see* Pindborg tumour
Cancer, 2, 5–7, 24, 77, 80, 114, 117, 119, 120, 122, 124, 126, 131–135, 138–142, 164
Carnoy's solution, 105–106, 156, 157
Cementoblastoma, 60, 68, 72, 82, 83, 90, 148
Cementum hyperplasia, 86
Chemotherapy, 33, 46, 114, 119, 122, 124, 126, 127, 130–132, 139
Cherubism, 50, 160
Chondrosarcoma, 44, 85, 123, 126
Clear cell odontogenic carcinoma, 113

D
Daughter cyst, 34
Dental follicle, 61, 152
Dentigerous cyst, 34, 36, 41, 55, 68, 94, 99, 151–154
Documentation, 14, 25

E
Epithelial cells rests of Malassez, 34
Ewing sarcoma, 123, 127
Excisional biopsy, 11

F
Fibrous dysplasia, 50, 83, 84, 91, 116, 137
Fine needle aspiration (FNA), 11, 12
Fixation, 13, 16
Formalin, 14–19, 23, 30

G
Giant cell granuloma, 50, 53, 63, 64, 70, 73, 75, 77, 90

H
Hemangiomas, 66, 118
Hematoxylin and eosin, 30
Hertwig's epithelial sheath, 34

I
Incisional biopsy, 11
Intraosseous, 7, 11, 12, 24, 49, 50, 53, 64, 79, 86, 97, 98, 111, 122–126, 130–138, 140, 160, 162

L
Leukoplakia, 6, 24, 25
Lichen planus, 6
Lymph nodes, 12, 88, 118, 125

© The Editor(s) (if applicable) and The Author(s), under exclusive license to Springer
Nature Switzerland AG 2024
N. Kochaji, *Clinical Oral Pathology*, https://doi.org/10.1007/978-3-031-53755-4

M
Median palatal cyst, 93
Mucoepidermoid carcinoma, 34, 66, 106, 127

N
Nasolabial cyst, 93
Nasopalatine cyst, 93

O
Odontogenic cysts, 97–111
Odontogenic ghost cell tumor, 113
Odontogenic glandular cyst, 76
Odontogenic keratocyst, 34, 35, 41, 47, 50,
        53–55, 58, 63, 68, 70, 72, 74, 93,
        99, 102, 103, 154–157, 160
Odontogenic myxoma, 28, 57, 68, 70, 72
Odontoma, 68, 73, 77–80, 82, 83, 90
Ossifying fibroma, 44, 45, 60, 72, 83, 90
Osteoma, 80, 83
Osteomyelitis, 50, 80–81, 87, 138
Osteosarcoma, 85, 123, 125

P
Paget's disease, 81, 91, 126
Paradental cyst, 57

R
Radicular cyst, 53, 55, 62, 94, 145, 148–151

S
Saline, 17–19
Simple bone cyst, 54–55, 66
Squamous cell carcinoma, 6, 25, 34, 50,
        66, 75, 123
Stafne bone defect, 66

T
Target therapy, 33, 139
Torus, 88
Transportation medium, 14
Traumatic bone cyst, 55

Periapical granuloma, 34, 55, 92, 146
Pindborg tumor, 91
Plasmacytoma, 93
Primary malignancies, 68, 121, 127
Primordial cyst, 41
Prognosis, 2, 4, 7, 25, 33, 34, 38–40, 44, 45,
        107, 111, 114, 119, 121, 122, 124,
        130, 131, 142, 151, 154, 157, 159
Punch biopsy, 11